UNSHACKLED

UNSHACKLED

Why Medicine Is Failing Doctors (and Patients)—and
How We Can Break Free

DR. HEATHER SKEENS

THIN LEAF PRESS | LOS ANGELES

Disclaimer—The advice, guidelines, and all suggested material in this book are given in the spirit of information with no claims to any particular guaranteed outcomes. This book does not replace professional consultation. Anyone deciding to add physical or mental exercises to their life should reach out to a licensed medical doctor, therapist, or consultant before following any of the advice in this book; anyone making any financial, business, or lifestyle decisions should consult a licensed professional before following any of the advice in this book. The authors, publisher, editors, and organizers do not assume and hereby disclaim any liability to any party for any loss, damage, or disruption caused by anything written in this book.

Library of Congress Cataloging-in-Publication Data
Names: Skeens, Heather, Author
Title: *Unshackled: Why Medicine Is Failing Doctors (and Patients)—and How We Can Break Free*
LCCN: 2025911109
ISBN 978-1-953183-98-9 (hardcover) | 978-1-953183-97-2 (paperback)
ISBN 978-1-953183-96-5 (eBook) | 978-1-953183-99-6 (audiobook)

Medicine, Healthcare & Work-Related Health
Cover Design: 100 Covers
Cover Photography: Rafael Barker
Interior Design: Dindo Sanguenza
Editors: Erik Seversen, Dhanliza Cellona
Thin Leaf Press
Los Angeles

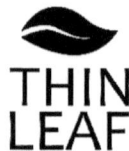

THIN
LEAF

This book is dedicated to all the doctors who have sacrificed their lives in service of others. May you find what makes your heart sing and the time to enjoy that before the end of your time here on this earth. And to Reid; the one who really made me a doctor.

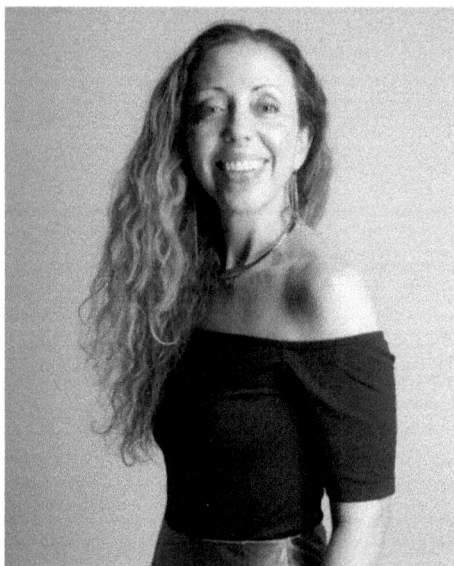

Dr. Heather Skeens, MD, CFMP, is a board-certified ophthalmologist, corneal transplant surgeon, and certified functional medicine practitioner who is redefining what it means to be a healer in modern medicine. As the founder of Bellasee™ Franchising, the first physician-owned ophthalmic franchise in the world, Dr. Skeens is leading a nationwide movement to restore autonomy, balance, and purpose to the lives of doctors—while bringing holistic, patient-centered care back to the forefront.

After years of witnessing both patients and physicians suffer under a broken healthcare system, Dr. Skeens combined her expertise in surgery, functional medicine, and entrepreneurship to create a revolutionary model that supports both healer and patient. Her journey is deeply personal, shaped by the tragic loss of her brother-in-law, Reid, and her own healing from autoimmune disease.

Dr. Skeens is also the founder of Bellasee™ Education, an online platform training physicians in new surgical techniques, remote clinic operations, and holistic health practices. Her work has empowered countless doctors to reclaim their careers and reimagine their lives.

She lives in Charleston, West Virginia, where she runs her flagship Bellasee™ Eyecare & Bellasee™ Skincare & Wellness practices. When she's not in surgery or mentoring other physicians, you'll find her writing, speaking, and continuing the work of building a better future for healthcare-one Bellasee™ clinic at a time.

Why Bellasee™ Matters

As you journey through the pages of this book, you will witness the raw and honest truth about the healthcare system: how it breaks doctors, betrays patients, and leaves both parties suffering in silence. But this book is not just a story of what is broken. It is a declaration of what can be rebuilt.

Bellasee™ is the movement I created out of necessity—a lifeline for physicians drowning in a system that was never designed to support their well-being, their autonomy, or their purpose. It is the first ophthalmic franchise in the world, but it is also so much more than a business model. Bellasee™ is an emancipation movement for doctors. It is a blueprint for a new kind of medicine—one rooted in compassion, integrity, and human connection. One where physicians are not employees of hospital systems, but owners of their own destiny.

To the physicians reading this: Bellasee™ is your "Get Out of Jail Free" card. It is your invitation to step out of the assembly line and return to the reason you became a doctor in the first place. We offer a real, tangible way to increase your income, reclaim your time, and practice medicine in alignment with your values.

To the patients reading this: there is hope. Bellasee™ is your alternative to the rushed, impersonal, bureaucratic system you've grown disillusioned with. It is where your doctor will know you. Where healing is the priority—not billing codes.

Together, we can change the future of medicine. But it starts with awareness. With courage. With you.

Join the Bellasee™ movement. Look for physicians and clinics who are part of it. Support them. Refer others. And if you are a doctor ready to make the leap, we are here, and we are waiting for you.

Learn more at www.bellasee.com.

Contents

Introduction

Why I'm Writing This Book

In the fall of 2024, something shifted in me. I began working with a spiritual mindset manifestation and business coach, and through this journey, I started uncovering truths about myself that had been buried beneath years of service, sacrifice, and survival. But to really understand why I'm writing this book; I need to take you back—seven years back.

Everything began to change in March 2018 when I learned that a very dear family member—my former brother-in-law, Reid—had been diagnosed with a rare form of cancer called sarcoma. At the time of his diagnosis, doctors told him he had just six months to live.

Reid was a private and deeply accomplished man. An attorney who spent most of his career advocating for children who had been abused or neglected, he lived a life devoted to helping others. At 54 years old, he appeared the picture of health—tall and lean at 6'1", active in the gym, conscious about his diet. Reid was also a free spirit. To say he marched to the beat of his own drum would be an understatement. Judges in court would delay his cases because they knew—if Reid wasn't present, he was likely off fishing. And they'd wait for him.

Every year, he would ride his Harley across the country, sleeping on the ground wherever he found a safe spot. He had a deep love for life, nature, and for people. He never met a stranger. Even those he prosecuted in court admired him. Though he never had biological children, Reid "adopted" many through international sponsorship programs, donating monthly. He truly was one of the good guys.

Reid met my sister when she was a student at the University of Kentucky. He was already practicing law. Fourteen years her senior, they had a complicated relationship—filled with passion, differences, reconnections, and heartbreak. Their marriage lasted about two years, but their connection endured far longer. In fact, hers was the last face he saw before his death. He always said his life began when he first saw her face, and he'd hoped hers was the last he'd see when it ended. He also said she was the only woman he could have ever married. And even after the divorce, Reid remained an integral part of our family.

When I learned about his diagnosis, I was devastated. I had experienced death before—as a physician, and through the natural loss of elderly grandparents and an aunt—but I had never faced losing someone so close, so young, and so suddenly. Reid's illness pulled me into a world I thought I already knew—medicine, mortality, care—but it turned out, I knew only the surface.

Over the next 1.5 years (Reid lived longer than he was expected, and I am going to tell you his story in this book; but not until you understand how his doctors were trained to treat him), I would become not just Reid's medical power of attorney and advocate, but his in-home hospice provider. I would become his witness. And through that experience—and through the world's sudden upheaval with the arrival of COVID-19 in 2020, just after Reid's passing — my entire perspective as a physician changed.

This book is about that change.

Through my work with Reid, I saw the brutal inadequacies of our healthcare system up close. I saw how doctors—people like me—are used as pawns in a system that exists primarily to benefit corporations, pharmaceutical companies, and insurance conglomerates. It became clear to me that we are voluntary slaves to a machine that feeds on our sacrifice. We serve, we give, and we lose ourselves in the process.

Doctors are no different than soldiers. We go into battle for others. We sacrifice our time, health, families, mental stability—for a calling we believe is noble. But what happens when the calling becomes a cage? What happens when the system we trusted starts to break us down?

Reid made me a doctor. Yes, I graduated from medical school in 2002. Yes, I passed all the exams. But it was Reid who made me a *physician*. Watching him face death with dignity, humor, and grace taught me more than any residency ever could.

And now, I write this book for every doctor who has ever felt lost in their own profession. I write it for the patients, too—so you might understand the human being standing in front of you in that white coat. So that you might pause and see the full journey it took to stand there and say, "How can I help you today?"

The past two years, especially, have been a time of deep reflection and inner transformation. Since November 2024, working with my mindset coach, I have been releasing old memories, blocks, and deeply ingrained patterns from my time in medicine. For the first time, I can see my true purpose clearly: I am here to help our doctors reclaim their lives. I want to help heal the healers.

This book marks the beginning of a paradigm shift in medicine— one where physicians reclaim control over their lives, their patients, and their purpose, breaking free from the quiet chains of voluntary slavery imposed by a system that was never built to serve them.

I didn't plan to write this book. I always imagined I might, someday. But I didn't plan to tell *this* story. It came to me like a wave— an undeniable urge I couldn't ignore. As I write, it doesn't feel like it's coming from me. It feels like it's coming *through* me. From a higher place. From the part of me that knows this message is needed.

So dear reader, I invite you to walk with me. Through the moments that shaped me. Through the heartbreak and revelations. Through the unraveling and rebuilding. This is my story—but it may very well be yours, too.

Reid: The Motorcycle

He took the same month off every summer—no itinerary, no companions, just the open road and his motorcycle. That was Reid. Quiet, observant, never rushed. He would pack light, toss a book or two in his worn leather bag (he loved reading), and disappear for weeks. He never called it "escaping," but I think it was.

Riding from sunup to sundown, he'd stop in small towns, strike up conversations with strangers at gas stations, leave generous tips at roadside diners. Sometimes he'd send us a postcard, but rarely. The world moved slower for Reid. Or maybe he had simply figured out something the rest of us hadn't.

He was the kind of man who remembered people's stories better than their names. A public service attorney by title, but in spirit, a philosopher. He lived simply, but intentionally. He donated anonymously, helped others quietly, and chose solitude not because he was lonely—but because that's where he found peace.

He was the kind of man that would show up on your doorstep unannounced, come in, and make himself home. He would laugh with your family, eat your food, make you feel like you were the most important person in the world to him at the time. He would share holidays and birthdays. Sometimes, if arriving in the middle of the night, he would sleep on your front porch, only to be found in the morning, not wanting to have woken you up.

Years later, I would learn that it was during one of those motorcycle trips that the first signs began. Subtle things. An odd rice-sized lump in his left thigh. But back then, none of us knew. Back then, he was just Reid on the road, chasing sunsets and breathing in freedom.

Before the hospitals.

Before the protocols.

Before the weight of it all.

There was just Reid.

And his motorcycle.

Chapter 1

My Journey into Medicine

I stumbled into a career in medicine. While many kids grow up knowing they want to be doctors—perhaps because they have a doctor in the family or parents who encourage them to be doctors—I had neither. I went to college thinking I would become a pharmacist. My uncle was a pharmacist, and when I was growing up, he was the only professional in our family. He was also the only person I had seen growing up who had real financial stability. He owned a nice house, drove nice cars, and always seemed to have enough money.

I grew up in the southern coalfields of West Virginia, in a small town called Williamson. Williamson, located in Mingo County—often referred to as "Bloody Mingo" due to its history—was best known for the infamous Hatfield-McCoy feud. Poverty surrounded me. The Williamson I knew was vastly different from the one people recognize today. Back then, it was a quaint small town, not yet consumed by the drug crisis. We had parades down the single main street for every holiday, and downtown was lined with small mom-and-pop businesses. There was a local shoe store, a clothing store, and a handful of other family-run shops.

Of course, I didn't buy anything myself—we didn't have money for extras. Every August, my aunt Dee Dee (Delores) took me school shopping at the one clothing store in Williamson. She made me try on what felt like a million pairs of jeans (an exaggeration, but it sure felt like it) until we found just the right pair. I also got a pair of penny loafers, as they were called back then. Fashion was never a consideration; practicality was. In December, I received more clothes to get me through the spring. Then, on my birthday in March, my grandmother—who was my wealthy uncle's mother—sent my sister and me a big box of clothes she had picked out. She had great taste, but again, we had no say in what we wore. Even as teenagers, we simply wore what we were gifted. We had no choice.

I was the oldest of my sister and me. Our parents divorced when I was four, and my father moved to Texas to work in the oil fields, where he had family connections. My father would remain an important part of my life growing up. Every June when school would let out, my mother would drive my sister and me to Tennessee to meet my dad and stepmother, who would then take us back to Texas with them until August, when it was time for school to start again. Then it was back to Tennessee to return us to my mom, and back to West Virginia. Back home, during the school year, my mother worked multiple jobs to provide for us—mainly as a secretary at a law firm during the day and at a shoe store at night. We had different babysitters until I turned 10; after that, we became "latchkey kids." We rode the bus home from school and let ourselves in with a key tied around our necks. We had neighbors across the street who we could go to in an emergency, but for the most part, we were alone until our mom came home from work.

Our street wasn't in the best neighborhood. It was lined with parked cars, and our yard was nothing more than a sliver of grass. Even as a child, before reaching my full height of 5'7", I could easily stand with both feet on concrete on either side of the grass. My sister and I played in the street, moving aside whenever a car came by. We rode bikes and roller skates—no helmets, no knee pads, just pure recklessness. There was one hill that still gives me chills when I think about how I skated down it. We couldn't even see the road below to check for oncoming traffic. What were we thinking? We were just kids having fun.

At the top of that hill lived an old farmer. I remember when he lost his thumb to a circular saw and had it replaced with his big toe. That freaked us out as kids, and we'd skate down the hill after reaching the top near his house, afraid of his "toe-thumb." Further up the street, there was another hill that led to a mountain path, which became our makeshift sledding hill in the winter. Of course, we didn't have real sleds—just garbage bags.

At the base of that path was a small grocery store where we occasionally bought candy. I still have dreams about that street.

The neighbors on one side of us were bad news. A woman lived there with her many sons—I don't remember how many. One of them, Butch, became a peeping Tom, watching my sister and me through our bedroom window while we got dressed in the mornings. We told our mom for weeks, but every time she rushed in, he had already ducked away. One day, he wasn't fast enough, and she caught him in the act. My mother, who had recently taken a handgun safety course at the police station, stormed outside with her gun and threatened to shoot him if he ever came near us again. He ran for his life. I truly believe she would have done it.

She had started taking those lessons after another one of the neighborhood boys, Greg Aleff, attempted to break into our house one night around Easter. Our home was separated from theirs by a narrow alley, leading to the back of our property and a garage entrance. Late one night, my sister and I saw Greg trying to open our bedroom window. We screamed for our mother, but she didn't believe us. It wasn't until he managed to pry open the wooden back door—only to be stopped by the chain lock—that she realized we weren't imagining things.

Panicked, she had us help her push a heavy counter against the door to keep him from breaking in. We could see his hand struggling to unlatch the chain from the outside. It was terrifying. I must have been 10, maybe 12. To this day, as an adult, I always keep my doors and windows locked.

When the police finally arrived, Greg had hidden in our garage. The officer found him, handcuffed him, and—strangely—brought him to our front door. My mother opened it with my sister and me clinging to her. The officer made Greg apologize. I still remember hearing, "Tell them you're sorry for what you did." Greg muttered a begrudging, "I'm sorry," and was taken away. He was released a few days later with nothing more than a restraining order. We were still terrified. And as it would happen, years later we would find out that Butch had been with Greg behind our house that night.

That experience made my mother determined to protect us, so when Butch started lurking outside our windows, he almost got his head blown off.

Moving to the City and Finding My Path

When I was 15, just before high school, my mother met my stepdad, and we moved to the "big city" of Charleston, WV. I enrolled at George Washington High School, and Williamson became a distant memory. Back then, high school was 10th–12th grade. Basketball became my saving grace. I had played since fifth grade and was already 5'7" by then— taller than most girls in my county. Basketball kept me grounded after moving to a new school where I knew no one. At George Washington High, I was suddenly surrounded by kids from wealthy families—kids whose parents were doctors, lawyers, and business owners. They had been groomed for success since birth. In contrast, my old town had very few wealthy families. Of the handful that existed, many of their children who did not make it out succumbed to drug addiction. There were other kids, of course, like me who did make it out and went on to have very successful careers for themselves. I think growing up the way we did in Williamson either made us strong and determined or had the opposite effect, forcing most to give up.

Ironically, at George Washington High, a still highly recognized National School of Excellence, eight students from my graduating class, including myself, went on to become ophthalmologists. But even in high school, I always felt like an outsider. When it came time to choose a college, I picked the University of Kentucky because they had the #3 pharmacy school in the country. I thought I would follow in my uncle's footsteps. He was the only person I knew who had money, so I figured that was the way to go. Then, one day, while walking between classes, I ran into a former high school classmate. We hadn't seen each other since graduation. I asked what he was studying, and he told me he was going to be a doctor—because there was no higher position than that. His parents were both doctors, and he believed that being a physician was the most respected profession one could achieve.

At that moment, I thought, *I want that. I want to be at the top.*

That day, I changed my major from pharmacy to biology and began my journey toward medicine.

Chapter 2

The Changing Landscape of Medicine: Then and Now

Looking back, it seems almost inevitable—common sense, even—that I would become a doctor. I have always taken care of others before myself. It's just who I am. Growing up in Williamson, West Virginia, along with the position of being the older sister, came responsibility. While my mother worked multiple jobs, I took care of my younger sister and helped manage the household. Now, as I raise my own children, who are 14 and 12, I'm struck by how young they still seem. At their age, I already felt like an adult. By seventh grade, I was cooking, cleaning, and ensuring my schoolwork was done—all while being the dependable person others could rely on. In ninth grade, I was voted "Most Likely to Succeed," not because I was the smartest, but because I worked hard and was responsible. I rarely played or goofed off. If someone had a problem, I wanted to fix it. If I couldn't, I genuinely felt like I had failed them.

Not too long ago, my mother showed me an old 1970s eye model that I used to play with as a child. I have no memory of it (doctors, as you will learn, have severe loss of memory due to years of sleep deprivation and chronic sympathetic nervous system overdrive), yet I wonder if it somehow shaped my path toward ophthalmology. I do remember the game *Operation*, which my dad got me for Christmas when it first came out. I found it oddly easy, removing the pieces from the tiny slots without ever setting off the buzzer. I couldn't understand why it was supposed to be a challenging game.

Unlike many doctors, my interest in medicine wasn't sparked by a family member's illness or personal experience with hospitals. Except for the one time my sister was hospitalized with near-fatal pneumonia and placed inside one of those bubbles, no one in my family was sick, and I rarely saw the inside of a hospital myself. I did break my pinky finger playing basketball in the street in seventh grade, which necessitated a trip to the emergency room. My journey to medicine wasn't about personal tragedy; it was about instinct, about responsibility, and perhaps, about always wanting to be the one who could fix things.

Medicine in the 1900s

The role of physicians in society has changed dramatically over the last century. In the 1920s and 1930s, doctors were revered as community pillars, trusted implicitly by their patients, and given full autonomy over their medical decisions. Medicine was a calling, not just a profession, and the doctor-patient relationship was deeply personal. Physicians made house calls, often knew multiple generations of a family, and their authority went unquestioned. We've all seen the movies where doctors are arriving in homes, sometimes on a horse and buggy if depicted in the 1800s, taking care of sick people. However, in the early 1900s, doctors' knowledge and resources were limited. Before the advent of antibiotics, many common infections were fatal, and doctors relied heavily on intuition rather than evidence-based medicine.

Ancient Wisdom Ignored—The Overlooked Influence of Eastern Medicine in the Early 1900s

While Western medicine in the 1800s and early 1900s was evolving rapidly through scientific discovery, sanitation practices, and the professionalization of the medical field, another entire world of healing existed—one that was largely ignored or misunderstood by U.S. physicians of the time. This was the world of Eastern medicine. It's important to clarify here: When I speak of "Eastern medicine," I'm not referring to individual healers from the East, but rather to the entire philosophy and framework of healing that originated in ancient civilizations such as China, India, and Japan. Systems like Traditional Chinese Medicine (TCM) and Ayurveda were not new in the 1900s—they were thousands of years old. These systems emphasized harmony, energy balance, and treating the root cause of disease rather than just the symptoms. An Eastern healer, then, was someone trained in these ancient traditions: someone who understood the body as an integrated system of energy (qi or prana), who used pulse diagnosis and tongue analysis to assess imbalance, and who viewed illness as the result of disharmony in one's physical, mental, emotional, or even spiritual life. Their toolkit didn't include surgical scalpels or synthetic drugs. It included acupuncture, herbal formulations, massage therapy (like Tui Na or Abhyanga), breathwork, dietary guidance, meditation, and movement practices like Tai Chi and yoga.

Many of the plant medicines used in Eastern traditions were virtually unknown to Western doctors in the early 20th century. For example:

- Astragalus root (used in TCM to boost immunity and vitality)
- Ashwagandha (an adaptogen in Ayurveda used for stress resilience and hormone balance)
- Turmeric/Curcumin (used for inflammation and detoxification)
- Licorice root (used in TCM to harmonize herbal formulas and soothe the digestive tract)
- Schisandra berry, reishi mushroom, holy basil, and many others

These were not folk remedies—they were part of documented medical systems that had been used successfully for millennia. Yet American physicians of the early 1900s had almost no exposure to these approaches. At best, they were dismissed as unscientific; at worst, ridiculed entirely. It wasn't until decades later, in the 1960s and 70s, that Eastern healing practices began to gain mainstream attention in the U.S. through the rise of integrative and holistic medicine. By then, pharmaceutical companies and insurance systems had already reshaped the medical landscape. Much of this ancient wisdom remained buried under a culture of clinical reductionism and industrialized care. What's astonishing is that many of the same herbs and plant-based therapies used in ancient Eastern medicine are now being validated by modern research for their effectiveness. But long before double-blind trials and peer-reviewed journals, these natural substances were already healing people. The sad truth is that American doctors—myself included—were not taught this history. We were not given the opportunity to understand what came before the stethoscope and the prescription pad. And because of that, we were robbed of tools that could have helped our patients and ourselves.

The Pharmaceutical Takeover: Contrasting 1900s U.S. Pharmacology with Ancient Eastern Herbology

In the early 1900s, U.S. pharmacology was entering a transformational phase. The prevailing model of medicine was shifting toward the identification and isolation of active compounds that could be standardized, patented, and mass-produced. This aligned with the scientific revolution of the time, but it also meant that more holistic, traditional approaches—including those rooted in ancient herbology— were sidelined or outright discredited. Western pharmacology focused heavily on symptom suppression and biochemical pathways. Synthetic derivatives of naturally occurring substances were favored because they could be patented and controlled. Willow bark, used for centuries to relieve pain, became aspirin. Mold spores led to penicillin. Opium became morphine. This was hailed as progress, and in many cases, it was life-saving. But there was a crucial difference: Eastern herbology had always used whole plants, often in combination, to achieve balance in the body—to simply to suppress one symptom at a time. For example,

Traditional Chinese Medicine (TCM) rarely used single herbs in isolation. Formulas were crafted with careful attention to how herbs interacted with one another and the patient's overall constitution. Ayurveda took a similar approach, treating the "dosha" imbalance behind illness, not just the complaint itself. This holistic view was incompatible with the reductionist, mechanistic framework that U.S. pharmacology adopted in the 20th century. American doctors were taught that herbs were "unscientific," even though nearly 25% of modern prescription drugs are derived directly or indirectly from plant sources.

The Rockefeller Influence and the Rise of Synthetic Pharmaceuticals

The sidelining of holistic and plant-based medicine in the U.S. wasn't just a byproduct of scientific evolution—it was also a calculated business strategy. In the early 20th century, John D. Rockefeller, one of the wealthiest men in American history, had a vested interest in promoting petroleum-based pharmaceuticals. Rockefeller owned Standard Oil, and through his investments in the pharmaceutical industry, he began to steer medical education and practice toward synthetic, lab-derived medicines that were dependent on petrochemical processes. In 1910, the Flexner Report, commissioned by the Carnegie Foundation and backed by Rockefeller's financial influence, restructured American medical education. The report declared that only allopathic (conventional, science-based) medicine was legitimate. As a result, hundreds of homeopathic, naturopathic, and herbal medicine schools were shut down or lost credibility. Funding was directed exclusively to institutions that followed the new pharmaceutical model. This marked a pivotal moment: plant-based and traditional medicines were marginalized, and synthetic drug development became the cornerstone of Western medical training and practice. Doctors were taught to prescribe pills—not to ask about food, emotion, movement, or energy.

And so, the wheel turned. Medicine became an industry, not a sacred art. And healing became a transaction.

From Autonomy to Algorithms: The Modern Physician's Dilemma

As the 20th century progressed, the physician's role transformed further. The Rockefeller influence marked the beginning of a new era in American medicine—one rooted in industrialization, standardization, and control. Over the following decades, medicine transformed from a noble calling and a healing art into a structured system of diagnostics, prescriptions, and insurance codes. And while this transformation brought remarkable advances in technology and treatment, it came at a cost.

Today, while Western medical advancements have vastly improved patient outcomes, the profession itself has lost much of its autonomy and societal prestige. Physicians are now subject to hospital administrators, insurance companies, and government regulations that dictate much of how they practice medicine. The doctor—the once-revered figure of wisdom and decision-making— has become an employee, in essence a voluntary slave, a data-entry clerk, and a procedural technician. The soul of medicine has been fragmented under the pressure of productivity metrics, billing codes, and bureaucratic oversight.

The Breaking Point: COVID-19 and Medical Autonomy

Perhaps no modern event better illustrates the tension between government control and medical autonomy than the COVID-19 pandemic. Amid uncertainty and fear, in 2021, the Biden administration, through the Centers for Medicare & Medicaid Services (CMS), implemented a federal rule requiring COVID-19 vaccination for healthcare workers in facilities that received Medicare or Medicaid funding as a condition of employment. This included hospitals, nursing homes, and outpatient clinics. For many physicians and nurses, this marked a turning point, not just in public health policy but in how medicine itself was governed.

Though some saw this as a public health necessity, many physicians, nurses, and frontline workers felt coerced into taking a vaccine they did not want, under threat of losing their jobs or medical privileges. Medical and religious exemptions were inconsistently granted. Clinical judgment was overruled by blanket policy. For those of us who questioned the long-term safety data, lacked trust in pharmaceutical influence, or had personal or medical reasons for hesitancy, the mandates were deeply unsettling, representing a loss of autonomy in a profession already stretched thin. Many of my physician and nurse colleagues lost their jobs because of refusing to take mandated vaccination.

This level of bureaucratic oversight—where government agencies superseded individual clinical decision-making—left many doctors feeling powerless. It reflected a broader trend: Medicine was no longer governed solely by evidence or ethics, but by politics, public pressure, and institutional liability. For a profession that had already suffered under increasing external control, the pandemic served as a magnifying glass. It exposed how deeply the autonomy of physicians had eroded—and how fragile that autonomy truly was when policy clashed with personal judgment.

Aftershocks of the Pandemic: Burnout, Shortages, and Eroding Trust

The COVID-19 pandemic didn't just strain hospital systems—it pushed the entire healthcare workforce to the edge. Long hours, emotional trauma, conflicting policies, and public scrutiny created a perfect storm of exhaustion. Physicians—already at risk for burnout before the pandemic—found themselves on the front lines of a prolonged, politicized crisis.

Burnout, which I'll explore more deeply later in this book, reached historic levels during the pandemic. Many doctors reported emotional numbness, moral injury, and feelings of betrayal by both institutions and the public. Healthcare workers were often placed in impossible situations—asked to follow constantly changing guidelines while facing personal risk, public skepticism, and overwhelming caseloads.

In addition to burnout, the system experienced a mass exodus of medical professionals. Nurses retired early. Physicians left clinical practice. Support staff were burned out or laid off. A survey by the Association of American Medical Colleges projected a shortage of up to 124,000 physicians by 2034—a shortage accelerated by the pandemic. Rural areas and under-resourced hospitals were hit especially hard. Perhaps most concerning of all was the shift in public trust toward medicine itself. Conflicting information from public health agencies, censorship of dissenting voices, and perceived politicization of science created deep divisions among patients.

Once trusted implicitly, the medical profession found itself questioned—sometimes rightly, sometimes from a place of misinformation and fear. The damage done to that sacred trust will take years, if not decades, to rebuild.

A Case Study in Dissent: Dr. Simone Gold and the Fight for Medical Freedom

For some physicians, the mandates were not just professionally disruptive—they were a call to action.

Dr. Simone Gold, an emergency medicine physician and attorney, emerged as one of the most visible critics of the government's pandemic response. As the founder of *America's Frontline Doctors*, she became a lightning rod for controversy by publicly challenging the safety, necessity, and ethical justification of the COVID-19 vaccine mandates. In a widely circulated video titled *The Truth About the COVID-19 Vaccine*, Gold voiced her deep concerns about the erosion of medical freedom and civil liberties during the pandemic.

In her address, Gold likened medical freedom to constitutionally protected rights such as speech and religion, arguing that no citizen, particularly no healthcare worker, should be forced into a medical decision under duress. She questioned the speed at which the vaccine was developed, the lack of long-term safety data, and what she described as an unprecedented level of coercion, not only from the government but also from institutional healthcare systems. Her central message was clear: Informed consent cannot exist in the shadow of mandates.

Gold's public dissent came at great personal cost. She was labeled as a conspiracy theorist in the media, faced legal consequences related to her involvement in political events, and was ultimately stripped of her ability to practice in many settings. Yet, to many like-minded physicians and patients, she became a symbol of resistance—someone willing to risk everything in defense of personal autonomy and the ethical practice of medicine.

Her story, like those of others who questioned the prevailing narrative, illustrates the high price of dissent in modern medicine. Dr. Gold represents a powerful example of a physician standing against what she viewed as government overreach, and in doing so, she reignited a broader debate about who truly governs the practice of medicine: the physician or the state.

Reinforcing Dissent: Robert F. Kennedy Jr. and the Institutional Critique

Dr. Simone Gold's concerns did not emerge in isolation. Public figures like Robert F. Kennedy Jr. echoed many of the same themes, raising deep skepticism about the interplay between pharmaceutical companies, public health institutions, and government mandates. In his book *The Real Anthony Fauci*, Kennedy details a troubling portrait of what he sees as systemic corruption at the highest levels of American health policy.

Kennedy argues that the COVID-19 response, particularly around the vaccine, was shaped less by transparent science and more by financial entanglements and conflicts of interest between regulatory agencies and the pharmaceutical industry. He points to Dr. Anthony Fauci's long-standing position at the National Institute of Allergy and Infectious Diseases as emblematic of a larger problem: a revolving door between federal oversight and industry profit. According to Kennedy, this convergence created an environment where dissenting voices were silenced—not because they were unscientific, but because they threatened profit models.

His book questions the unprecedented power given to a few individuals during the pandemic and critiques the blanket application of mandates, regardless of natural immunity, risk profile, or personal health status. He argues that such policies violated basic principles of informed consent and bioethics, undermining the autonomy not only of patients, but also of physicians trying to make individualized decisions.

Kennedy's concerns bolster the argument that the pandemic became a moment of reckoning—not just for medicine, but for democracy itself. Physicians like Dr. Gold weren't just resisting a vaccine; they were resisting a system that no longer allowed questions. For those of us who felt the weight of that system during the pandemic, Kennedy's research and documentation provided intellectual validation for a truth we had already begun to feel: When public health becomes politicized, medicine loses its soul.

My Stand: A Physician's Personal Decision

Like Dr. Gold and Robert F. Kennedy Jr., I, too, came to a deeply personal decision during the pandemic—one that placed me at odds with the very system I was trained in. Despite my conventional education as a medical doctor, I refused the COVID-19 vaccine. This was not a decision made in haste or rebellion, but one rooted in years of clinical observation, personal medical history, and an unwavering belief in the body's innate ability to heal. I had a strong conviction that my immune system could withstand the virus. I had never received viral vaccinations in the past, and I saw no reason to treat this virus any differently. More importantly, I have a history of autoimmune disease—something I had worked tirelessly to put into remission. To introduce a foreign agent that could potentially disrupt that delicate balance felt reckless and irresponsible, especially given what I knew through both traditional and functional medicine training.

Just prior to the pandemic, I had emerged from the trauma of watching my loved one, Reid, suffer through the brutal failures of conventional cancer care. There was simply no way I was going to place my trust—let alone my body—into the hands of a system that had failed us so profoundly. My refusal came with consequences. After seven years of faithfully serving a rural community, I was forced to resign my surgical privileges at one of the outpatient centers I had long operated in. They denied my medical exemption. Thankfully, the main hospital where I also performed surgeries accepted a religious exemption and allowed me to continue. Living and practicing in a conservative state like West Virginia proved to be a blessing. Many of my patients and colleagues felt similarly disillusioned by the mandates. The sense of solidarity gave me the courage to remain true to my convictions.

What troubled me most, however, wasn't just the mandates—it was what I began to see in my own patients. I noticed an alarming uptick in corneal transplant rejections following COVID-19 vaccination. Some of these rejections occurred in patients whose transplants I had performed a decade earlier, patients who had never shown signs of immune response or instability. We've long known that certain vaccines, like influenza, can occasionally trigger graft rejection due to the immune system being stimulated into overdrive. But these COVID-related rejections were different. Unlike typical rejection episodes, which can often be reversed with a regimen of topical, oral, or even subconjunctival steroid injections, these grafts failed to respond. Vision was lost, and repeat transplants were needed. The timing, the severity, and the non-responsiveness were impossible to ignore.

Even more concerning were the cases where patients received multiple vaccinations—COVID-19, influenza, and pneumococcal—on the same day, per their primary physician's advice. From my perspective as a corneal surgeon, this wasn't informed care. It was graft suicide.

Footnote:

[1] Reports have documented cases of acute corneal graft rejection following seasonal influenza vaccination, particularly in patients with penetrating keratoplasty. The proposed mechanism involves immune activation and inflammation following immunization.

[2] Emerging case reports and small studies have identified a potential temporal association between COVID-19 vaccination and corneal graft rejection. Although causality is still under investigation, clinicians have observed immune-mediated rejection episodes occurring shortly after mRNA vaccination, particularly in stable grafts with no prior history of complications.

I Stayed Open

Beyond the institutional failures and the political noise, the pandemic forced an even more personal reckoning. For me, and for many doctors like me, the crisis wasn't just unfolding in headlines or hospital policy memos. It was happening in real time, in our clinics, in our homes, and in our hearts. The tension between duty and mandate, between science and conscience, had never been so palpable. What I didn't expect was just how much it would challenge the core of my identity as a physician. The very ground I had stood on for decades, the sacred promise that no matter the chaos, I would always be able to serve—suddenly felt like it was being taken from me.

As a physician, I had always taken comfort in one fundamental truth: No matter what was happening in the world, I would always be able to serve. I knew how to care for people. That was my purpose, and it was my security. Through every challenge in medicine, that knowledge—that I could always help someone—grounded me. But during the COVID-19 pandemic, something shifted. For the first time in my life, I was told by the government that I could not do my job. That as a physician, I was to close my doors, cancel care, and go home. Not because I lacked training, resources, or courage, but because policymakers with no medical degrees and seemingly no calling to heal had decided that physicians like me were no longer "essential." I remember feeling a deep helplessness. And more than that, a profound sense of injustice. How could those who had never taken an oath to serve, who had never stood at a bedside or held a hand through suffering, be given the authority to silence the healers? I had built an independent outpatient ophthalmology clinic with my own hands, and I was a corneal transplant surgeon. My patients depended on me—some had fresh transplants, others were losing vision, in pain, afraid, and without options. And yet I was told to abandon them. But I couldn't. I wouldn't.

Despite pressure from professional boards and government mandates, I made the decision to keep my clinic open. Every day, I feared I would be shut down. Every day, I worried I might lose my medical license. But my patients came first. They always had. Patients with painful infections, failing grafts, progressive disease—they couldn't wait weeks or months for care. And I couldn't bear to leave them without it. I was not reckless. I was prepared. My training in both conventional and functional medicine (I had my degree in functional and integrative medicine by that time, too) gave me a deep understanding of the immune system. I had confidence in my own health, nutrition, and resilience.

Like many physicians, I had spent years exposed to countless viral and bacterial illnesses, and my immune system was strong. I knew how to protect myself and my patients. But more importantly, I knew that not showing up for them would violate the very core of who I am as a doctor. To be told I could not care for people felt, in many ways, like being told I could no longer breathe. It was as if someone had told a mother her child was sick, but she was not allowed to go to them—even though she had the medicine in her hands. That pain, that separation from purpose, is something I struggle to put into words, and I know many doctors felt the same.

And so, I made my choice. I stayed open. I kept working. And though I lived with the daily fear of retribution, I did so willingly—because my patients needed me. And I needed to be there for them.

A Fractured Relationship

The experience of being silenced during the pandemic opened my eyes to a deeper fracture within our healthcare system—one that extends far beyond clinic walls. It was not just the mandates that were troubling; it was the realization that the sacred bond between doctor and patient, once rooted in trust and mutual respect, had started to erode. The public began to question our motives, our decisions, and even our compassion—not because they no longer needed us, but because something more insidious had taken root in the background. The rise of digital media, social networks, and sensationalized headlines created a landscape where misinformation thrived, and fear spread faster than any virus.

The Media Frenzy and Viral Vaccines

The COVID-19 pandemic did not just challenge our physical health systems—it triggered an unprecedented information crisis. Media outlets, once considered reliable sources of public health information, became battlegrounds of fear, speculation, and politicized narratives. From 24-hour cable news to viral Twitter threads, the noise was deafening and dangerously inconsistent. Every day brought conflicting messages: stay home, go out, wear a mask, masks don't help, the vaccine is safe, the vaccine is rushed. For the average patient, it became nearly impossible to discern fact from fearmongering. What made this even more perilous was the speed with which misinformation spread. A single post, often unverified, could reach millions in hours, undermining decades of evidence-based medical guidance and sparking widespread public confusion.

The introduction of the COVID-19 vaccines became another flashpoint. For many physicians, it was a moment of pride-proof of what modern medicine could achieve. But for the public, flooded with polarized media commentary and conspiracy-laced social media content, the rollout raised more questions than answers. Rather than unifying communities around public health, the vaccine narrative often deepened mistrust, especially as mandates and passport requirements were introduced without clear, consistent explanations. This constant media pressure not only sowed distrust among patients—it also placed physicians in the crossfire. We became unwilling messengers of politicized policies, often bearing the brunt of public anger for decisions we did not make. As we attempted to educate and reassure our patients, we were met with skepticism fueled not by reason, but by headlines, hashtags, and viral videos. It was heartbreaking. Our patients needed us more than ever, but many no longer knew whether to trust us.

Reid: The First Signs

It had been a while since I'd spoken to Reid. The last time I saw him was that Easter, a year prior to his diagnosis, just before he and my sister set off on an Alaskan cruise with friends—one of their many attempts to give love another try.

They were in that in-between space again. Reid had moved back in with her, back into the house they once shared in Ashland, Kentucky. It was familiar territory, but time hadn't softened their differences. My sister is structured, tidy, and regimented. Reid—well, Reid was Reid. Free-spirited. Drifting in his own rhythm. They both loved hard, but in different directions.

Still, they had their moments. Long walks, often for hours. Workouts together at the YMCA—the same place they had first met, decades ago, in the University of Kentucky's weight room. They cooked together, too. He'd tease her endlessly about her "health food," never knowing if her latest dish was meant for humans or dogs. Once, he pulled what he thought was a homemade cookie from her countertop jar—only to learn too late it was one of her dog's biscuits. He still finished it. Said it tasted weird, but figured it was one of her protein-packed, low-sugar experiments. We laughed about that one for years.

Reid took care of her dogs when she worked late at the hospital. He loved listening to her stories about the psychiatric patients she counseled. He called her job heroic. He meant it. Despite all the reasons they couldn't quite live together, he admired her deeply.

But the cruise broke them.

Too much closeness. Too many hours boxed in together, floating somewhere between the glaciers and their own emotional icebergs. She wanted space. He wanted to roam. A ship, in hindsight, may have been the worst place for them to test their bond.

After that, the calls stopped for a while. Life moved on. Or at least I thought it did.

When he finally called me again, something was off. His voice sounded strange. He sounded anxious in a way I didn't recognize. He didn't sound like Reid. It was almost Christmas. He said he wanted to talk to me about LASIK eye surgery. I urged a meeting in my office to evaluate him. He said he would be back in touch. He was feeling tired. He'd seen someone—urgent care, maybe, he didn't really say—that he needed to follow up with and he'd let me know.

It would be months before I learned it wasn't.

Chapter 3

The Calling to Medicine: A Journey of Passion and Perseverance

Doctors do not enter medicine for the money. If you ask any physician, medical student, or resident why they chose this path, their answer will likely revolve around a fascination with the human body and an unwavering desire to help people. Of course, there are those whose parents force them into medicine. But these are not as many as you would think. In all my years in the medical field, I have never heard a doctor say, "I went into medicine for the money." The reality is, if financial gain were the primary goal, there are far easier and less demanding career paths.

Becoming a doctor is a calling—one that few truly understand before embarking on the journey. We enter medical school driven by an innate need to heal, but with little understanding of the sacrifices required. Perhaps some are drawn to the prestige or the idea of performing surgeries, much like the dramatized portrayals on shows like *Grey's Anatomy* (though I must point out that when they depict ophthalmologists performing eye surgery, it's painfully obvious they're working on a cow or pig eye rather than a human one).

For me, ophthalmology was not an initial aspiration, but rather, it was a path illuminated by a mentor. The summer before starting medical school, I needed a job, and through a connection, I began working as a scribe for an ophthalmologist in my hometown of Charleston, WV. I knew nothing about eyeballs, but I threw myself into the role with determination. On my first day, after observing my work, the doctor called me into his office. I thought he was about to fire me. Instead, he gave me an unexpected raise, saying I had exceeded his expectations. From that day on, he took a vested interest in my learning, bringing me into every patient encounter and teaching me about various eye conditions. He even taught me how to use an ophthalmoscope—an invaluable tool for looking into the back of the eye. At the end of the summer, he gifted me my first ophthalmoscope, a gesture that symbolized his belief in me.

That man changed my life. I still remember calling him in a panic on my first day of medical school, terrified and uncertain. He reassured me, calming my nerves in the way only a great mentor can. From that moment on, I knew; I was meant to be an ophthalmologist.

The importance of mentorship within the field of medicine cannot be overstated. Doctors are mentors to each other in ways that shape careers, character, and confidence. Many medical students and residents choose their specialties because of the influence of a compassionate, inspiring attending mentor who took the time to teach and lead by example. Beyond training, physicians continue to guide and mentor one another through shared experiences, clinical challenges, and emotional burdens. We are not only teachers to medical students but also to nurses, staff, and even our patients. Medicine is a collective effort, and we rely on each other more than we often admit.

Before my summer scribing experience, and before deciding on ophthalmology, I had considered radiology. During college, I shadowed a radiologist at the University of Kentucky and found the field fascinating. But ophthalmology had everything I wanted: a perfect blend of clinical practice and surgery (I did like working with my hands), manageable hours compared to a general or trauma surgery field, and compared to these surgical fields, the potential for a work-life balance that would allow me to raise a family. Most importantly, I was captivated by the eye itself. The first time I looked into someone's eye with a magnifying lens, it felt like stepping into another world—a private, intricate universe visible only to me. The eye is an extension of the brain, and examining it offers a glimpse into the body's neural network. I remember thinking, *"Wow, I really can see into their soul!"*

The Reality of Becoming a Physician

Knowing you want to be a doctor is only the first step. The road to becoming one is an entirely different battle. Getting into medical school is no easy feat. It takes years of preparation, an impeccable academic record, and relentless determination. To even be considered, you must be at the top of your college graduating class, complete rigorous pre-med coursework, and endure the relentless scrutiny of your GPA.

Envision a young mind, bright and unclouded, fueled by curiosity and compassion. This is our young, wannabe doctor. A college student who wakes up early to study while the campus sleeps, driven not by the arrogant or narcissist ego they will be accused of eventually having, but by a deep yearning to help. Their world is still full of possibility—untouched by cynicism, unshaped by systems. They volunteer in hospitals, shadow physicians, and stay up late poring over biology textbooks, imagining the day they'll wear a white coat of their own. Their whole life revolves around this one dream: to rise to the top, not for status or wealth, but to alleviate suffering, to heal, to matter. It's a kind of beautiful naivety—a pure-hearted belief that through knowledge and service, they can make the world better.

I don't remember college as a time of socializing or carefree fun. While others went out on weekends, I was grinding, studying day and night. At the University of Kentucky, the only events that ever pulled me away from my books were basketball games at Rupp Arena. Basketball was the one sport I understood well, having played from fifth grade through high school. In 1998, the year I graduated, UK won back-to-back national championships, first in '96 and then in '98. I remember that season vividly. Kentucky hasn't won a national championship since. But outside of those occasional moments of escape, my focus was singular:

29

getting into medical school. I only applied to a handful of programs, including Kentucky and Marshall and West Virginia Universities—the two schools in my home state. When I received my rejection letter from UK, I remember how much it stung. It wasn't a simple "we regret to inform you" notice. Instead, it was a long-winded explanation about how many people apply, how not everyone is cut out for medicine, and how they just didn't believe I had what it took to be a doctor. They suggested I pursue a different career path. I saved that letter somewhere. Someday, I hope to find it again. I fear it may have been lost in a house fire during my first year of ophthalmology residency, when everything I owned was reduced to ashes. This was before cell phones made it easy to capture every moment, but I still have a vivid memory of that letter in my mind. I laugh every time UK's ophthalmology department sends me a referral. I laugh when patients from between Charleston, West Virginia, and Lexington, Kentucky, are given the choice to travel to me for cornea care or to go to UK, and they choose me, even when I'm farther away. Don't get me wrong, UK has an excellent ophthalmology department. I know because my stepsister is a pediatric ophthalmologist there. But they rejected me not once, but twice. After medical school, I applied to UK for my ophthalmology residency, and again, they declined my application. Maybe I had some deep need to prove that I could make it despite their doubts. Maybe I wanted validation. But looking back, it worked out exactly as it was meant to, because I had no intention of attending their program.

Getting into medical school is difficult at best. Many students who want to be doctors do not get accepted into a program. As of the most recent data from the Association of American Medical Colleges (AAMC), for the 2023–2024 application cycle, 55,188 students applied to U.S. allopathic (MD) medical schools, 22,981 students matriculated, meaning over 32,000 applicants were rejected or did not gain admission that cycle. This means approximately 58% of applicants did not get accepted into a U.S. MD medical school.

Medical School: Tests, Trials, and Tenacity

Getting into medical school requires more than a great GPA. There's the Medical College Admission Test (MCAT), a standardized test that can determine a doctor's future in medicine before they've even set foot in a medical school classroom. The MCAT is a standardized, computer-based examination designed to assess problem-solving, critical thinking, and knowledge of natural, behavioral, and social science concepts and principles prerequisite to the study of medicine. It is administered by the Association of American Medical Colleges (AAMC) and is required for admission to medical schools in the United States, Canada, Australia, and the Caribbean Islands.

The MCAT is widely regarded as one of the most challenging standardized tests in existence, due to its broad scope and emphasis on analytical reasoning. Students dedicate months and often years preparing for this exam while balancing their studies with undergraduate coursework, clinical experiences, and research.

A competitive MCAT score is not just a requirement; it is often a determining factor in securing admission to a top-tier medical school. Even with this, medical schools consider the MCAT just one piece of the admissions puzzle. Candidates are also evaluated holistically based on academic performance, extracurricular involvement, clinical experience, and personal qualities essential for a career in medicine.

Volunteer work in a hospital environment or medical clinic is expected as well. I, for example, volunteered in the emergency room of my local hospital the summers of my sophomore and junior years of college, and then in the radiology department at UK for a semester during the school year. The emergency room was where I first had exposure to real trauma. Vivid recollections of a man with full-body third-degree burns from a gasoline explosion; the sight of him writhing in pain; the smell of his burning flesh, all vivid in my mind. The patients ejected from cars, not wearing seatbelts, limbs torn apart. The motorcycle and four-wheeler trauma patients with no helmets worn, paralyzed now. It's a lot to take in for a young woman in her early 20s.

These weren't scenes from a TV drama. These were real lives, real suffering, and they deeply shaped my drive to serve. They also started my journey into a life of Post-Traumatic Stress Disorder (PTSD), something most doctors will suffer from at some point in their careers. PTSD is a mental health condition triggered by experiencing or witnessing a traumatic event. It can lead to persistent emotional distress, intrusive memories, and physical symptoms that disrupt daily life. I will explore in Chapter 5 how PTSD manifests uniquely in physicians—often in silence—and why this conversation is long overdue.

The Illusion of Supply: Rising Interest, Worsening Shortages

Medical school is a four-year crucible: two years of classroom science and two years of hospital rotations. Over the years, the number of premedical students applying to medical school has fluctuated, reflecting shifts in societal attitudes and broader changes within the medical profession.

In 1998—the year of my college graduation—approximately 41,000 students applied to U.S. medical schools, marking a period of relative stability in application volume. At that time, medicine was widely viewed as a prestigious and stable career path, consistently attracting individuals drawn to its purpose and promise.

In recent decades, there has been an uptick of interest in the medical field, but this does not necessarily guarantee an adequate supply of practicing physicians. By 2025, the number of medical school applicants is projected to exceed 60,000—a sharp increase from previous decades. Several factors are responsible for this surge, including the expansion of medical sub-specialties, increased awareness of global health issues, and the establishment of new medical institutions that have broadened access to training opportunities. These trends underscore the continued demand for physicians and highlight how shifting educational dynamics continue to shape the aspirations of future doctors.

Despite rising application numbers, however, the United States is facing a significant shortfall of medical professionals. According to projections by the Association of American Medical Colleges (AAMC), the nation may experience a shortage of between 37,800 and 124,000 physicians by the year 2034—an alarming gap that spans both primary care and specialty services.

In the field of ophthalmology specifically, a notable workforce shortage is anticipated by 2030. This looming deficit can be attributed to several intersecting factors: an aging population requiring more eye care services, a large portion of the current ophthalmologist workforce nearing retirement, and a limited number of residency training slots that restrict the entry of new specialists into the field. These projected shortages make clear the urgent need to improve working conditions and foster a more sustainable environment for current practitioners— while also ensuring the field remains attractive and accessible to future generations of doctors.

Reid: And Cancer

When I first learned Reid had cancer, I didn't pause. I didn't cry. I didn't sit with the grief or even process what it meant. I just wanted to fix it.

That instinct, so deeply wired into me from years of training, years of responsibility, took over completely. Reid had cancer. They hadn't told him what type at this point. Just said a rare, aggressive form. And all I could think was: What can I do? Who can I call? Where do we start?

He sounded calm when he told me. Too calm. I could tell he was trying to protect me—trying to make it easier somehow. But behind his even tone, I could hear the weight settling into his voice. The way people sound when they're holding back a storm.

I went into doctor mode. Started researching, reading every article I could find, reviewing clinical trials, case reports, anything. I sent emails to specialists I didn't even know at every major cancer center across the United States. I called in favors. My entire focus narrowed to one goal: get Reid well. I stopped eating and sleeping. If I wasn't taking care of my patients or my boys, I was working for Reid.

It wasn't about being heroic. It wasn't about being right. It was about not letting someone I love fall through the cracks I had seen so many patients disappear into. I had been trained to manage sickness, to perform surgeries, to keep people functioning, to restore eyesight. But this was different. This was someone I loved. Someone who trusted me now more than ever.

For the first time, medicine wasn't just my profession. It was personal.

Chapter 4

The Cost of Becoming a Doctor

Getting into medical school is hard. Paying for it is even harder. Most doctors take out loans, and I was no exception. I didn't have a wealthy family to fund my education. I vividly remember my grandmother telling me that medical school was too expensive and that I should pursue something else. She had no idea how I planned to pay for it, and that was my clue that I could expect no financial support from my family. But I didn't care. I had paid for my undergraduate education through loans, scholarships, and working odd jobs whenever I had time. During my first few years at UK, I didn't have a car. I walked everywhere, across a sprawling campus that seemed to stretch endlessly. My grandmother wasn't wrong to worry about the cost. She had no idea how long it takes to pay back medical school debt or how little doctors earn in residency. But instinctively, she understood something that most people don't: There are much easier ways to make a living.

Medical school tuition is staggering. Remember this tuition is following the tuition paid to attend a four-year college where the aspiring physician is studying for the MCAT and obtaining a required undergraduate degree. As with college tuition, staying in-state helps— tuition is about half the cost of out-of-state—but even then, the numbers are daunting. When I attended as an in-state public medical student, tuition was around $20,000 per year—it is now closer to $45,000 per year. Those attending a public medical school out-of-state face significantly higher costs, with median tuition and fees reaching $66,000. These figures emphasize the financial advantages of remaining in-state for medical education as out-of-state students often pay nearly 50% more for the same degree.

Tuition costs can also vary widely depending on whether a student attends a public or private institution. The cost of medical education is a crucial consideration for aspiring physicians as it plays a major role in student debt accumulation and long-term financial planning. In contrast to an in-state, out-of-state comparison, private medical schools have a standardized tuition structure regardless of residency status. The median tuition and fees for first-year students at private institutions are $72,689, making them the most expensive option overall. Unlike public schools, private medical schools do not offer reduced tuition rates based on residency, further increasing the financial challenges for students who choose this path.

It is important to note that these figures only represent direct costs associated with tuition and mandatory fees. Additional expenses including health insurance, living costs, textbooks, and educational materials further contribute to the overall financial burden of medical school. Doctors, while they are college graduates, are not being paid a salary to attend medical school and often need to take out loans above and beyond those required for tuition and books to have money to pay rent and eat.

Starting a Career in a Financial Hole

Aspiring doctors do not enter medicine for money, but ironically, money becomes an overwhelming factor in their journey. Medical education in the United States is one of the most expensive academic pursuits, leaving most students saddled with staggering debt before they even begin practicing. The escalating cost of medical education has become a significant concern, with the median education debt for medical school graduates reaching approximately $200,000 as of 2019. Keep in mind this does not include any remaining college education debt. And doctors cannot deduct the interest we pay on student loans when doing taxes—per the government, we make too much money to do so.

This substantial financial burden influences medical students' career choices, often steering them toward higher-paying specialties to manage their debts effectively. Unlike other professions where higher education debt is at least somewhat balanced by an immediate, well-paying job, newly minted doctors enter residency earning a salary between $30,000 and $65,000 per year for the subsequent three to seven years—hardly enough to quickly pay off their loans, especially after years of delayed income.

In addition, medical school tuition is just one piece of the financial burden. Other hidden costs add up quickly. Applying to residency programs costs hundreds to thousands of dollars and traveling for interviews can add another few thousand. The USMLE exam series (a grueling three-step series designed to test medical knowledge and clinical decision-making during medical school and residency) is costly. Step 1 alone is over $600, and Step 2 and Step 3 come with their own hefty fees. Even after residency, physicians must pay thousands for board certification exams and renewal fees every few years. After 20 years of practice, I still pay annual board certification dues to maintain board certification. In addition, once in practice, doctors must carry malpractice insurance, which can cost anywhere from $10,000 to $200,000 annually, depending on the specialty.

By the time a doctor is fully licensed and practicing, they may be in their mid-30s and will work to pay off loans for a large portion of their career. Compare this to peers who entered other fields right out of college, many of whom have been earning, investing, and buying homes for a decade while physicians were still training. This financial burden isn't just stressful—it's a major factor in why many doctors reconsider their career path.

After four years, upon completion of medical school, doctors enter residency, where they train under grueling conditions for an additional three to seven years depending on their specialty. The financial landscape for medical residents has seen minimal growth over the past two decades, failing to keep pace with escalating educational costs and inflation. Between 2002 and 2006, when I was a resident, residents typically earned approximately $30,000 annually. In 2023, the average resident salary was reported at $67,400, reflecting a 5% increase from the previous year's $64,200. While this nominal increase suggests progress, when adjusted for inflation and considering the rising costs of medical education and living expenses, the real income growth for residents remains relatively stagnant.

The disparity becomes more pronounced when considering the demanding work hours associated with residency programs, which often extend up to 80 hours per week, and in some cases approach 100 to 120 hours per week. This workload translates to an approximate hourly wage of $16 to $20, if just 80 hours are worked, at a pay of $67,400 annually, raising concerns about fair compensation for the labor-intensive nature of medical training. Geographical location further influences the financial well-being of residents. States offering higher salaries, such as California and New York, also contend with elevated living costs, effectively diminishing the purchasing power of these increased wages. Conversely, regions like the Southern United States report average PGY-1 salaries around $60,514, which, although lower, may offer a more favorable cost-of-living balance.

To summarize, the cost of medical school has nearly tripled in the last few decades, but resident salaries have remained essentially frozen in time. The equivalent of what I earned in residency is what I now pay my front desk receptionist, who works 40 hours a week at $19 per hour. Residents, on the other hand, and for example those earning $60,000 per year, often work 80 to 120 hours per week, which means in some cases, they are making even less than minimum wage. This is a person who has completed four years of college, four years of medical school, and is now holding a professional degree as a doctor, performing procedures, making life-or-death decisions. Yet they are paid less than a fast-food worker. Worse yet, if we assume 120 hours per week, the pay comes out to less than 10 dollars per hour. Even if a resident "only" works 80 hours per week, they are making $14 per hour for an entire year, without a single week of paid vacation. And holidays? Forget it. While contracts state allowed vacation and holiday time, in reality, residents don't get Christmas off. They don't get Thanksgiving with their families. They work through birthdays, anniversaries, even the birth of their own children. I equate this to the "optional" Saturday basketball practices my sons have on their middle school basketball team. Everyone knows you can take the "option," but in doing so, you pay a penalty.

Chapter 5

Residency -Where the Real Indoctrination Begins

It's not just about getting into medical school and paying for it; once you're in, you must excel. Your performance determines which specialty you can pursue, and for competitive fields like ophthalmology, you must be at the top of your class. Graduating medical school doesn't mean you can practice medicine. You must "match" into a residency—a multi-year, full-time training position in your chosen specialty. The match process is complex and expensive. Applicants rank programs, programs rank applicants, and a computer determines placement.

This is not a simple application process—it's a high-stakes, costly endeavor. During their fourth year, medical students apply to dozens of programs, with some submitting applications to as many as 50 or more. Each application costs money, and the more programs you apply to, the higher the financial burden. I, perhaps naively, applied to only seven. Fortunately, I matched at my in-state program, the WVU Eye Institute. But many students are not as lucky. For those who don't match, the options are grim: Either wait another year to reapply, hoping to strengthen their application, or pivot to a different specialty with open positions. There's also the *Supplemental Offer and Acceptance Program* (SOAP), a frantic, last-minute scramble where unmatched applicants apply for unfilled residency spots. Some ultimately must choose a less competitive specialty or reconsider their entire career trajectory.

And that's just residency. Before even reaching that stage, medical students must pass the United States Medical Licensing Exam (USMLE). Step 1 is taken after the second year of medical school and focuses on basic sciences like anatomy, biochemistry, pathology, and pharmacology. It was once a numerical score but has now become pass/fail—though that does little to lessen its importance. Step 2 is typically taken during the fourth year and assesses clinical knowledge and hands-on skills. It includes a component where students must diagnose actors posing as patients. Step 3, the final hurdle, is taken during residency and evaluates whether a doctor can practice independently. It includes both multiple-choice questions and computer-based patient simulations. Failing any of these exams can derail a medical career entirely. Passing them is merely a requirement to continue the grueling climb.

The Real Purpose of Residency

Residency is not only training into a specific branch of medicine. Residency is designed to groom doctors into believing that their only purpose on this earth is to serve others, especially the healthcare system and Big Pharma, at any cost, without expecting fair compensation. If we ever question the "standard of care," attempt to explore alternative therapies with our patients, dare to ask for better pay, if we ever suggest that we, too, deserve to be financially compensated for our work, we are called greedy, selfish, and accused of not caring about our patients. Residency is not just training; it's indoctrination. We learn to prioritize service over self, to accept exhaustion as normal, and to believe that questioning the "system" is selfish and career suicide.

Residency is also a period of profound influence, where the culture of modern medicine is imprinted on young physicians. While we are taught to diagnose with precision and intervene quickly, the deeper art of healing—understanding why a person is sick in the first place—is often overshadowed. Instead, we are encouraged to match symptoms to pharmaceuticals, to see illness as a list of codes and prescriptions rather than a human story.

Residency turns doctors into voluntary slaves.

Pharmaceutical Influence in Medical Training

This way of thinking doesn't begin in residency—it starts in medical school. Bright-eyed and burdened with debt, we are inundated with free lunches and glossy pamphlets from pharmaceutical representatives who pose as friendly guides. Their presence is so normalized that many students barely question the ethics of it. Yet behind the catered meals and casual conversations is a clear agenda: shape our prescribing habits early and often. One study found that 100% of surveyed medical students reported some form of interaction with the pharmaceutical industry, with 65% receiving gifts or meals, and over 50% believing that these interactions did not influence their behavior—even though studies show otherwise. Another study found that pharmaceutical companies spend over $20 billion a year marketing to doctors in the U.S. In 2009, the Institute of Medicine published a landmark report titled *Conflict of Interest in Medical Research, Education, and Practice*, which exposed how financial relationships with pharmaceutical and medical device companies were compromising the integrity of medical training and clinical care. The report concluded that even seemingly small gifts or financial ties could influence prescribing behaviors and clinical decisions—often unconsciously. It called for sweeping reforms, including full transparency in physician-industry relationships and a cultural shift away from industry-sponsored education.

I recall one of my colleagues from medical school entering the field of primary care medicine; in his outpatient clinic, he refused to allow pharmaceutical-sponsored lunches or even allow pharmaceutical representatives in his clinic in the first place. This colleague was 20 years my senior as medicine was his second career. He had a deep knowledge of the influence pharmaceutical companies can have on a doctor, even as a fresh medical school graduate first entering clinical practice. The rest of us did not have this understanding at the time. Sadly, this physician and classmate of mine would pass away a few years later from Lou Gehrig's disease. He was a tremendous doctor and IronMan athlete. He had also been a professional ballerina in his former life prior to medicine, but when I think about him today, I remember him for the stance that he took against the pharmaceutical industry.

The result of pharmaceutical influence is a subtle but powerful conditioning. Doctors are trained to see drugs as solutions rather than tools, symptoms as targets rather than signals. Over time, this shapes not only our practice but our identity as physicians. The deeper question of "Why is this person unwell?" gets lost in the noise of symptom checklists, formularies, and performance metrics.

If we are to reclaim the soul of medicine, we must start by questioning who shaped our training, and why. Healing begins with truth, and the truth is, much of our education has been sponsored by those who profit from our prescriptions.

The Emotional and Physical Toll of Training

Medical training isn't just expensive—it is emotionally and physically grueling. From the first day of medical school, students are thrown into an environment of intense competition, sleep deprivation, and relentless expectations. The academic pressure alone is overwhelming. Medical students must memorize volumes of complex medical knowledge, much of which will never be directly useful in practice but is nonetheless required for exams. By the time a medical student has learned medical terminology, they have learned an entire new language. The "sink or swim" mentality is deeply ingrained, and failure is not an option. Every test, every grade, every step of the way matters for future career prospects.

Following completion and graduation from medical school comes residency. Residency is where the real physical and emotional toll begins. The long hours are infamous—many doctors work 80 to 100 hours per week, often on minimal sleep. The concept of a "24-hour shift" is not a myth.

The stress extends beyond just the hours worked as well. The demanding nature of the medical profession has long been associated with high levels of stress, burnout, and, tragically, increased rates of suicide among physicians. A critical, yet often underemphasized factor contributing to these issues is sleep deprivation. Sleep is not optional. It is the body's primary healing mechanism—physiologically, emotionally, and spiritually. According to the U.S. Centers for Disease Control and Prevention, lack of sleep increases the risk of chronic diseases like diabetes, hypertension, depression, obesity, and even cancer. It reduces productivity, erodes quality of life, and impairs cognitive function. But sleep isn't just about energy restoration. It's when the body detoxifies. It's when tissues repair. It's when the brain processes and purges undigested emotions, experiences, and stressors that we couldn't metabolize during the day.

Sleep is sacred. It's not simply a break from productivity—it's medicine. And yet, in conventional medical culture, sleep is the first thing we sacrifice. Doctors are trained to wear sleep deprivation as a badge of honor, not realizing that in doing so, they are slowly dismantling their own health from the inside out. The rigorous schedules that many doctors endure frequently lead to insufficient rest, which can severely impact their mental health and overall well-being.

I completed medical school in 2002, residency in 2006, and fellowship in 2007. Those years were grueling. Residency tested the limits of human endurance. I worked over 100 hours a week—sometimes up to 120. We would start our shifts in the morning, work through the night, and continue into the next day. Only then after a 48-hour stretch were we allowed to go home and collapse—just to wake up and start all over again. Call shifts were brutal. I wasn't even in general surgery or OB/GYN, yet as an internal medicine resident, I was constantly on my feet. Sleep was a luxury we were rarely granted. Nurses and emergency room staff paged us nonstop to handle medical situations, no matter how exhausted we were. I remember feeling so tired that I was physically ill. There was no time to eat, and when we did, we were left with hospital cafeteria food that had little to no nutritional value.

The effects of sleep deprivation extend beyond immediate cognitive impairments; they also have profound implications for emotional regulation. Research indicates that inadequate sleep disrupts the brain's ability to manage emotions effectively, leading to increased irritability, anxiety, and depressive symptoms. Notably, sleep loss has been shown to amplify emotional reactivity, making individuals more susceptible to negative moods and stressors. I recall being made to watch a movie in medical school on the detriments of sleep deprivation. A mother was depicted in the movie, working days at a time with no sleep. She had both daytime and nighttime jobs. She also had a baby. After five days and nights without sleep, her baby crying endlessly through the night, the mother killed her own child just to get a quiet place to sleep. I have forgotten a lot of things that happened during my medical training—remember, doctors have issues remembering lifetime events—but I remember this movie as if I were watching it now. It was horrifying. The point they were trying to make is that sleep is so important for human brain function, that our brains will direct us to perform whatever action necessary to get it, even if it means killing your own child. Ironically, we were then not given the choice to make sleep a priority. And, despite our relentless sleepless schedules, as students and residents, we were expected to always maintain a cheerful demeanor. If we showed even the slightest frustration with a nurse or another staff member, we risked being reprimanded by our attending physicians. Too many strikes, and you could be thrown out of the program.

Chronic sleep deprivation has been linked to structural and functional changes in brain regions responsible for mood regulation. These alterations can impair decision-making abilities and increase impulsivity, factors that may elevate the risk of suicidal ideation among sleep-deprived individuals. Sleep deprivation among physicians is thus more than just an inconvenience—it's a dangerous threat to mental health. Physicians are already at elevated risk of depression, burnout, and emotional fatigue, and chronic sleep loss only magnifies these issues. The emotional toll of long shifts, overnight call, and minimal recovery time can push doctors past their breaking point. Tragically, this has led to a disproportionate rate of suicide in the medical profession. One large-scale analysis found that 17% of physicians reported suicidal ideation, and approximately 1% had attempted suicide. Female physicians, in particular, are at significantly higher risk—with suicide rates up to four times higher than their non-physician counterparts.

Recent studies have further highlighted the prevalence of sleep deprivation among healthcare professionals. For instance, a survey conducted by the Medical Defence Union (MDU) revealed that one in three NHS doctors reported that extreme tiredness had impaired their ability to treat patients, with 26% acknowledging that their patients had been harmed or experienced near misses as a result. This alarming statistic underscores the direct correlation between lack of sleep and compromised patient care, further exacerbating the stress and guilt experienced by physicians. In addition, the persistent lack of restorative sleep not only hinders physicians' professional performance but also poses a serious threat to their mental and physical health. For doctors, who regularly face high-pressure situations, heightened emotional sensitivity from a lack of sleep can contribute to burnout and a diminished capacity to cope with the demands of their profession.

Studies show that sleep-deprived physicians have cognitive impairment comparable to a person with a blood alcohol level of 0.08% (the legal limit for intoxication). Doctors are expected to put patients before themselves. Self-care is a foreign concept during residency. There's no time to eat properly, exercise, or even take restroom breaks on busy shifts. Looking back, the irony is glaring: doctors—the very people responsible for teaching others how to care for their bodies—are themselves deprived of the most basic necessities of health: sleep, nutrition, and rest. It is an impossible expectation, which can lead to devastating consequences with patients. Unlike other professions where errors may be fixable, medical mistakes may have life-or-death consequences. Mistakes can mean patient harm—or even death. This constant pressure can be crushing. And let's not forget the emotional trauma doctors experience in taking care of patients. Doctors witness suffering, death, and difficult conversations with families daily. Many specialties, particularly emergency medicine and intensive care, come with high exposure to trauma.

PTSD

Post-Traumatic Stress Disorder (PTSD) is a psychiatric condition that arises following exposure to traumatic events, leading to significant disturbances in an individual's cognition, emotional regulation, and behavior. Symptoms often include intrusive memories, avoidance behaviors, negative alterations in mood and cognition, and heightened arousal. For a diagnosis of PTSD, these symptoms must persist for more than a month and cause substantial distress or impairment in daily functioning.

In the medical profession, the prevalence of PTSD varies notably across specialties. Emergency physicians, for instance, have a point prevalence of approximately 15.8%, significantly higher than the general U.S. population's rate of 3.8%. During the COVID-19 pandemic, family medicine physicians exhibited PTSD rates of 31.2%, while emergency medicine physicians had rates of 23.4%. Among medical trainees, such as interns, 10.8% screened positive for PTSD by the end of their internship year, a rate three times higher than the general population's 12-month prevalence.

The onset of PTSD symptoms typically occurs within three months following a traumatic event; however, there are instances where symptoms may emerge after a delay of months or even years. Once established, PTSD can become a chronic condition, with symptoms persisting for months or years, and in some cases, leading to lifelong challenges.

When comparing medical professionals to combat veterans, it's evident that both groups are at heightened risk for developing PTSD due to their exposure to traumatic situations. While combat veterans face life-threatening scenarios in war zones, physicians often encounter severe injuries, patient deaths, and high-stress environments, especially in specialties like emergency medicine and surgery. The prevalence rates of PTSD among physicians in certain specialties are comparable to, or even exceed, those observed in combat veterans, underscoring the profound impact of medical practice on mental health.

Despite the significant prevalence of PTSD among physicians, mental health issues have historically been stigmatized within the medical community. This stigma often discourages healthcare professionals from seeking necessary mental health care, fearing professional repercussions or being perceived as weak. Such attitudes can exacerbate the severity of PTSD symptoms and hinder recovery. Recognizing these challenges, various resources have become available to support physicians dealing with PTSD. Peer support programs, confidential counseling services, and institutional wellness initiatives aim to provide safe avenues for medical professionals to seek help. Additionally, organizations like the American Medical Association and Physicians Anonymous offer resources and support networks to address mental health concerns within the profession. However, many states still require physicians to disclose mental health histories when applying for medical licensure. These questions can deter physicians from seeking treatment due to concerns about licensure implications. While the intent is to ensure patient safety by identifying impaired practitioners, overly broad inquiries may infringe on physicians' privacy and discourage them from addressing their mental health needs. Efforts are ongoing to balance the necessity of assessing physician competence with the imperative to promote mental well-being among healthcare providers.

In conclusion, PTSD presents a significant concern within the medical community, with prevalence rates varying by specialty and often mirroring those found in high-risk populations like combat veterans. Addressing this issue requires a multifaceted approach, including reducing stigma, providing accessible mental health resources, and reevaluating licensure processes to encourage physicians to seek the help they need without fear of professional repercussions.

Burnout

Residency is supposed to be temporary, just a steppingstone to independent practice. But for many, it is the breaking point. Burnout begins early, and the consequences extend far beyond residency. Burnout is defined as a state of emotional, mental, and often physical exhaustion brought on by prolonged or repeated stress. Physician burnout is more than just exhaustion; it is a full-scale crisis that threatens the very foundation of modern medicine. The word "burnout" is thrown around casually, but in the medical profession, it represents something far more dangerous. It is not simply feeling overworked or drained at the end of the day; it is a relentless, chronic depletion of emotional, physical, and mental well-being. It is the kind of exhaustion that does not go away with a vacation. Left unchecked, it leads to disengagement, depression, and, for far too many, suicide.

The numbers paint a grim picture. Over 60% of physicians report experiencing burnout. Suicide rates among doctors are among the highest of any profession, with an estimated 300 to 400 doctors dying by suicide each year in the United States—an entire medical school class, gone, every year. Women physicians are twice as likely to die by suicide as their male counterparts. Nearly half of all medical residents experience severe burnout before their careers even begin. This is not just an individual problem; it is a systemic failure. A profession built on healing is now destroying the very people it relies on to keep others alive.

Burnout is defined by three key symptoms. Emotional exhaustion drains doctors to the point where they feel they have nothing left to give. Depersonalization sets in, making it difficult to connect with patients, reducing them to cases rather than human beings—a coping mechanism for the unrelenting emotional toll of medicine. Finally, a diminished sense of personal accomplishment leaves physicians questioning whether their work even makes a difference.

For some physicians, burnout becomes the catalyst for radical reinvention. They don't just leave a job—they leave the entire system. One such example is Dr. Mira Shah.

Dr. Mira Shah, a board-certified family physician turned certified functional medicine provider, knows this reality firsthand. After years of working in federally qualified health centers and high-pressure primary care roles, she hit a breaking point. Burned out and disillusioned, she left traditional medicine. The final straw came after she was physically assaulted by a patient—a trauma that left her with severe PTSD. With no real institutional support, she walked away from the system and began designing a life that worked for her and her family. Today, Dr. Shah runs her own clinic where she picks up her kids from school, sets her own hours, and sees patients on her terms. "You do make less money," she says, "but it's much better. I'm in charge of my schedule. I'm not dictated by a hospital or group. I take care of patients the way I want to."

Dr Shah's story is not isolated. The following are additional examples of physicians who have stepped away from traditional models of care—not out of weakness, but out of necessity. Each of these doctors reached a point where the system no longer served their patients, their families, or their health. What they chose instead were new paths built on autonomy, purpose, and healing. Their stories remind us that there is another way—and that the future of medicine may be written not by institutions, but by the bold individuals who dare to walk away and begin again.

Real Stories: The Human Cost of Physician Burnout

Numbers and statistics paint a bleak picture of burnout, but the reality is even more devastating when you hear the voices of real physicians—those who entered medicine with passion, only to be broken by the system. These are their stories.

Dr. Sarah L., Emergency Medicine: "I Became a Machine, and I Didn't Even Recognize Myself Anymore."

Sarah was the type of doctor every patient wanted. Compassionate, thorough, and dedicated. She went into emergency medicine because she loved the adrenaline, the fast-paced problem-solving, and the ability to save lives in critical moments. But over time, the system crushed her. Her shifts were relentless—14-hour days, no real breaks, no food, no water, and barely a moment to breathe. She watched patients sit in hallways for hours because there were no beds. She saw colleagues crack under the pressure—some turning to alcohol, some leaving medicine altogether. She stopped sleeping. "I used to cry in my car before my shift—not because I didn't love medicine, but because I knew what was waiting for me: a never-ending line of suffering people I couldn't help the way I wanted to." Then one day, she found herself doing chest compressions on a 9-year-old girl who had been in a car accident. The child didn't make it. Sarah went home that night and stared at her reflection in the mirror. She realized she felt nothing. "I had become a machine. No emotions, no grief, no joy. Just numb. That scared me more than anything." She left emergency medicine a year later. She now works in telemedicine—a far cry from the ER, but it allows her to still practice without destroying herself. She still mourns the loss of the doctor she used to be.

Dr. Mark R., Internal Medicine: "I Gave Everything to Medicine, and It Took Everything from Me." Mark was a devoted internist, one of the few primary care doctors who truly took his time with patients. He believed in medicine the way it should be practiced—thoughtfully, with deep relationships and comprehensive care. But medicine today doesn't allow that. Insurance companies dictated how much time he could spend with each patient—15 minutes, no more. If he wanted to do a thorough job, it meant staying late to finish hours of charting. He spent more time fighting insurance denials than actually helping people. "I started realizing I wasn't a doctor anymore. I was a data-entry clerk, pushing buttons in an electronic medical record system that was never designed for patient care—it was designed for billing." His wife noticed the changes first. He stopped exercising, stopped laughing. He would come home late and collapse into bed, too exhausted to eat dinner with his kids. Then the chest pains started. At first, he ignored them—he had too many patients to see. Then one day, he collapsed in the middle of clinic. A heart attack. He was 42 years old. "The irony wasn't lost on me. I spent my life teaching patients about self-care, yet I was the one who almost died from stress." That was his wake-up call. He left full-time practice and now teaches at a medical school, helping train the next generation. But he warns them: "This system will eat you alive if you let it."

Dr. Emily T., Surgery: "I Loved Surgery, But Surgery Didn't Love Me Back." Emily was one of the few female surgeons in her field. She had always been drawn to the precision and artistry of surgery, and she worked harder than anyone to prove herself. But surgical training was brutal. "As a woman, I felt like I had to be twice as good, twice as tough, and never show weakness." She prided herself on being able to push through exhaustion. She would go 48 hours without sleep during residency, then head straight into the OR for a 10-hour case. Her breaking point came on a holiday weekend. She had been working non-stop, running on caffeine and adrenaline, when her hands started shaking during an operation. She almost made a critical mistake. "For the first time in my career, I had to step away from the table. I had never felt so ashamed." That night, she sat in her car for over an hour, sobbing before she could even go inside. She had given everything to surgery, but it had given her nothing in return. She eventually left hospital-based surgery and transitioned into outpatient surgical practice, where she could set her own schedule. But she still struggles with guilt. "I feel like I walked away. But if I had stayed, I don't think I'd be alive today."

Dr. James P., Psychiatry - "Even as a Mental Health Doctor, I Couldn't Save Myself." James entered psychiatry to help others navigate their mental health journeys. He believed deeply in supporting patients through depression, anxiety, and trauma. But he didn't expect to struggle himself. His patient load was overwhelming—30 or more people a day. Insurance companies routinely denied the medications he knew his patients needed. Suicide rates among his patients were rising, and he felt powerless to stop it. He began having panic attacks before work. He would sit in his car, gasping for air, knowing he had to face another day of suffering he couldn't fix. "I knew all the signs of depression. I knew I was heading into the abyss. But I felt like I couldn't ask for help. Who helps the helper?" One night, after a particularly devastating patient suicide, he went home and pulled out his own bottle of pills. He almost ended his life. A close friend intervened, and he was able to begin therapy. He now advocates for physician mental health, but he remains haunted by how close he came to becoming a statistic himself. "We tell our patients to seek help. But we don't feel safe doing the same."

The Human Cost of a Broken System

These stories are not isolated. They are repeated thousands of times over—across every specialty, in every hospital, and every clinic. Physicians are trained to be strong. But they are still human. And right now, the system is breaking them. How many more doctors do we have to lose before real change happens?

Physician suicide rates are staggering yet rarely discussed. Male physicians are nearly one and a half times more likely to die by suicide than the general population, and female physicians are at even higher risk. Medical students and residents, some of the brightest minds in the world, are already drowning in depression before they have even started their careers. And still, the system refuses to acknowledge the depth of the crisis. Physicians don't just take their lives because they are tired. They take their lives because they feel trapped in a profession that has stripped them of their humanity. They take their lives because they see no way out.

The doctor who once found deep fulfillment in healing now wonders if they are just another cog in the machine. The root of this crisis is not simply long hours—doctors have always worked long hours. The difference now is the increasing loss of control over how medicine is practiced. The doctor-patient relationship, once the heart of medicine, has been reduced to a series of bureaucratic hurdles. Physicians enter medicine to care for people, but instead, they spend their days trapped behind screens, buried under endless documentation, prior authorizations, and administrative red tape. Over 50% of a doctor's workday is spent on paperwork. For every hour spent with patients, two more are consumed by clerical work.

The joy of medicine has been buried under an avalanche of digital checkboxes, hospital metrics, and insurance constraints. Doctors have become data entry clerks, trying to satisfy hospital administrators while patients are rushed in and out like products on an assembly line.

The calling to heal has been hijacked by a system that prioritizes profits over care. The grueling work hours only exacerbate the problem.

Physicians do not get the luxury of an off switch. On-call duties can mean 36-hour, or worse, 48-hour shifts without sleep. Surgeons may operate for 12 or more hours straight without a break to eat, drink, or even use the restroom. Even so-called regular clinic days can stretch into 14-hour marathons between patient visits, charting, and follow-ups.

Sleep deprivation is a direct cause of medical errors, yet the system continues to demand superhuman endurance from its doctors. Imagine a pilot being asked to fly a plane after being awake for 36 hours or 48 hours straight. That would be unthinkable. But we expect doctors to do the same, with human lives in their hands.

The pressure to be perfect is relentless. Medicine is one of the only professions where one mistake can end a career, cost a life, or result in a lawsuit. Over 75% of physicians are sued at some point in their careers, often not because of actual negligence, but because bad outcomes happen even when doctors do everything right. The fear of litigation forces physicians to practice defensive medicine, ordering unnecessary tests and procedures just to protect themselves legally. This hyper-critical, zero-error expectation places enormous mental strain on doctors who are already stretched beyond their limits.

Despite all of this, there remains a suffocating stigma around physician mental health. Doctors are trained from the start to push through exhaustion, stress, and trauma. The culture of medicine reinforces the idea that self-care is selfish, that admitting struggle is weakness. Many physicians avoid seeking help because they fear it will be seen as a sign that they are unfit for the profession. In some states, physicians who disclose a history of mental health treatment can be denied a medical license or required to submit to invasive investigations. The result? Doctors suffer in silence. Many turn to alcohol, prescription medications, or isolation instead of seeking professional help. This isn't just burnout; it's moral injury. Doctors are being forced to practice medicine in ways that violate their ethics. They are rushed through patient visits when they know proper care requires more time. They watch insurance companies deny essential treatments they know their patients need. They are overruled by hospital executives who see patient care as a financial transaction rather than a moral obligation. Doctors do not simply burn out; they are broken by a system that no longer values what they do.

But this crisis is not inevitable. Burnout is not a personal failing; it is the result of a broken system. If we want to keep our best doctors, if we want to save the future of medicine, we need real change. The stigma around physician mental health must end. Doctors should be able to seek help without fear of losing their licenses or being seen as unfit. The crushing administrative burdens must be lifted so that doctors can spend time with patients instead of being buried under paperwork. The healthcare system itself must be restructured so that patient care, not profit, is the priority. Work-life balance must be a standard, not a privilege granted only to those who can afford to step away. Physicians dedicate their lives to healing others. It's time we start healing them, too.

Impostor Syndrome in Physicians

Impostor syndrome, also known as impostor phenomenon, is a psychological pattern in which individuals doubt their accomplishments and persistently fear being exposed as a "fraud" despite evident success and competence. First identified by psychologists Pauline Clance and Suzanne Imes in 1978, this internal experience leads individuals to attribute their achievements to luck, timing, or external help rather than their own ability.

In medicine, impostor syndrome is remarkably common, particularly given the high-stakes, high-performance environment in which physicians operate. Many physicians, from medical students to seasoned practitioners, experience the feeling that they are not as competent as others perceive them to be. This can lead to chronic self-doubt, overworking, burnout, and even avoidance of career advancement opportunities.

Studies suggest that approximately 30% of physicians experience symptoms of impostor syndrome at some point in their careers. This rate may be even higher in early-career physicians, residents, and those in academic medicine. The syndrome is exacerbated by the culture of perfectionism in medicine, where mistakes are feared, and vulnerability is often stigmatized.

Recognizing and addressing impostor syndrome is essential not only for the physician's well-being but also for cultivating healthier work environments and improving patient care outcomes. As awareness grows, medical schools and hospitals are increasingly offering wellness programs, mentorship, and psychological support to help physicians combat impostor thoughts and build confidence in their clinical skills.

Doctors as Voluntary Slaves

The real truth is doctors are trained to be voluntary slaves. We enter medicine with the noble goal of helping others, only to find ourselves trapped in a system that demands total sacrifice. Every day, we put our lives on the line, exposing ourselves to blood, feces, spit, and disease, enduring verbal abuse, working until our bodies give out. Our sympathetic nervous systems are stuck in overdrive, releasing cortisol 24/7, leading to chronic inflammation, gray hair, skin disorders, digestive problems, and premature aging. And yet, we are expected to always perform at peak levels. Because if we make one mistake, one human mistake, we can be sued, fired, or have our entire career destroyed. We are talked down to by our superiors in training, sometimes belittled by our patients, and treated as disposable by the institutions we work for. And when we do get paid, the money is thrown at us with a silent warning: Don't ask for another dime.

The combination of soaring educational debt and stagnant, inequitable salaries contributes to physician burnout and dissatisfaction, potentially exacerbating the anticipated physician shortage. Addressing these financial challenges is crucial to ensure the sustainability of the healthcare workforce and to maintain high-quality patient care. Honestly, I could have owned a plumbing or construction company and made more money than I have as a doctor.

Reid: The System

It took nearly a month just to get an appointment.

Johns Hopkins. One of the most prestigious names in medicine, and yet the wait felt like an eternity. By the time Reid sat across from the oncologist, nine months had passed since he first started chasing a diagnosis. It wasn't until the Hopkins pathology team re-reviewed the old samples that the truth finally came to light: sarcoma. Rare. Aggressive.

I'll never forget the way they said it—clinical, detached. They told us the medications wouldn't cure anything. That the treatment would, at best, buy him a little time. Maybe. There was no plan for wellness. No curiosity. No questions about how he was eating or sleeping. No questions about his mental state or spiritual life. Just scans. Just protocols. Just tumor measurements.

They didn't see Reid.

They didn't know that he was still coughing up blood and driving himself to Cleveland for treatment—alone or with a work friend who didn't ask questions. They didn't know he still wore a suit to court. That he still tried to work every day. That he shaved his head preemptively so no one would see him lose control of anything—not even his hair.

They didn't ask. And Reid didn't offer.

He was that kind of man. He never wanted to burden anyone. He said he was okay. That if this was God's plan, he was ready. His only fear was incapacitation—not death. Just the slow erasure of who he was. He told me, "I don't want to be here if I can't be me." I believed him.

But I wasn't ready to give up. I couldn't. I didn't hear, "There's nothing we can do." I heard, "We haven't found it yet." I refused to believe this was the end. Not for Reid. Not for someone so alive.

What broke me was how little they tried. Heads down. Notes scribbled. Eyes on scan reports instead of the man sitting right in front of them. I was watching medicine—the profession I had given my entire life to—fumble the most basic thing: seeing the person.

He wasn't a chart. He wasn't a timeline.
He was Reid.
And they missed him entirely.

Chapter 6

Where Is the Money Going?

If physicians are paid so little during their training, and patients struggle to access to care, where is all the money in medicine going? Medical schools and hospital systems in the United States generate substantial annual revenues, derived from various streams such as patient care services, research grants, tuition, and philanthropic contributions. These institutions serve as the backbone of the healthcare system, funding cutting-edge research, training the next generation of physicians, and providing critical medical services to communities. However, while these institutions command immense financial resources, concerns have arisen regarding how these funds are allocated, particularly in relation to physician salaries, patient care investments, and executive compensation.

According to the Association of American Medical Colleges (AAMC), U.S. MD-granting medical education programs with full LCME accreditation reported total revenues of approximately $192 billion in fiscal year 2023. Of this, $105.5 billion (54.9%) was recorded directly on medical schools' financial books, while the remaining $86.6 billion (45.1%) was managed by affiliated entities such as hospitals or practice plans. Similarly, hospital systems command enormous financial resources. The American Hospital Association (AHA) reports that there are 6,093 hospitals across the United States, with large hospitals (those with more than 250 beds) experiencing an average annual net revenue increase of 6.2% between 2018 and 2022. These figures highlight the immense financial influence of medical institutions, yet physicians, especially those in training, see little of these revenues reflected in their salaries.

How is Funding Distributed?

Despite these substantial revenues, funding is not evenly distributed across the healthcare system. A significant portion of these funds is allocated toward patient care services, covering costs associated with direct patient care, medical supplies, and facility maintenance. Another significant expenditure is research and education as institutions invest heavily in scientific research, clinical trials, and training programs for future physicians. Administrative expenses also consume a large share of these revenues as salaries for hospital executives and management teams continue to rise. And this is where the questions start coming into play.

Executive compensation in nonprofit hospital systems and medical institutions has become a particularly controversial topic. Some of the highest-paid executives earn multimillion-dollar salaries, raising concerns about financial priorities within the healthcare industry. For example, in 2021, Madeline Bell, CEO of the Children's Hospital of Philadelphia (CHOP), received a total compensation package of $7.7 million, making her one of the highest-paid children's hospital executives in the country. Similarly, executives at Ascension Health, a major nonprofit healthcare organization, have received annual compensation exceeding $10 million. At the University of Pittsburgh Medical Center (UPMC), top executives also receive multimillion-dollar compensation packages, reflecting the institution's extensive revenue streams.

The scale of these executive salaries has sparked widespread debate, particularly given that many of these institutions operate under nonprofit status, benefiting from tax exemptions while physicians, particularly those in training, struggle with stagnant wages and increasing workloads. Meanwhile, patients face rising healthcare costs, often unaware that a significant portion of hospital revenues is funneled toward administrative salaries rather than direct patient care.

Medical schools and hospital systems undoubtedly require significant funding to operate effectively, supporting research, medical education, and patient care. However, the disproportionate allocation of funds—where hospital administrators and executives command multimillion-dollar salaries while doctors experience wage stagnation and patients struggle to pay for needed services—calls into question the financial priorities of the healthcare system.

Hospital Funding and Profitability During the Pandemic

During the COVID-19 pandemic, the U.S. government allocated substantial funds to support hospitals facing unprecedented challenges. These financial interventions had varied impacts on hospital profitability and raised questions about the equitable distribution of aid.

In response to the financial strains imposed by the pandemic, the U.S. government introduced relief measures, notably the Coronavirus Aid, Relief, and Economic Security (CARES) Act. This act provided significant financial assistance to hospitals to offset revenue losses and increased operational costs. Studies indicate that these relief funds contributed to record-high profit margins for many hospitals during 2020 and 2021. For instance, a report by Mathematica and the National Academy for State Health Policy highlighted that median net profit margins for hospitals rose to their highest levels compared to prior years, fueled by federal and state COVID funding.

Similarly, an analysis published in *JAMA Health Forum* revealed that hospital operating margins reached an all-time high during the first two years of the pandemic. The study suggests that COVID-19 relief funds allowed some hospitals to achieve top financial performance rather than merely addressing financial solvency.

Disparities in Fund Distribution

Despite the overall financial bolstering of hospitals, the allocation of relief funds was not uniform across all institutions. Research indicates that academic-affiliated hospitals and those with higher pre-pandemic assets received more substantial funding, while critical access hospitals, often serving rural communities, received comparatively less financial assistance. This disparity suggests that relief funds may have disproportionately benefited hospitals that were already in a stronger financial position before the pandemic.

Profits at the Top, Pressure at the Bottom

While government relief bolstered many hospital systems during the pandemic, the financial windfalls were not felt equally across the healthcare workforce. In fact, the same institutions that received generous federal support and recorded record profits often failed to pass those benefits on to the very physicians who sustained the system under extraordinary pressure. Physicians remain burdened by student debt, stagnant pay, and an increasing administrative workload. This growing imbalance between institutional profitability and frontline physician well-being has revealed a deeper fracture where the business of medicine continues to thrive, even as the people practicing it are burning out.

And while physicians are bearing the weight of a broken system from the inside, patients are suffering just as deeply on the outside—trapped in a structure that too often puts profit before people. It's a painful irony: In one of the wealthiest nations in the world, patients are skipping medications, delaying care, or walking away from prescriptions at the pharmacy counter, not because they don't need them, but because they can't afford them. I've watched patients break down in my exam chair, not because of their diagnosis, but because they knew they couldn't pay for the treatment. We prescribe hope, and insurance companies deny it at the register. Every day I am questioned after discussing a treatment option needed to restore eyesight: "Will this be covered by my insurance?" Or I am told on a follow-up visit, after my care plan was not followed, and the patient has suffered: "That medicine you prescribed was $600, I can't afford that."

Patients are embarrassed to call me after a trip to the pharmacy to say they could not get the medication—so much so that they will suffer the disease process as an alternative.

I have personally experienced this with a topical medication that I use on my skin occasionally when my psoriasis lesions flare. This medication was quoted at over $1,200 monthly with my health insurance coverage at the pharmacy. I was able to find the same medication produced in Canada for $125 and order it from Canada pharmacy online once a year when needed.

My staff and I spend countless hours submitting prior authorizations and answering questions regarding the need for the prescribed treatment, and why they cannot have the insurance suggested alternative.

Cornea transplant rejection provides a prime example. One of the most potent topical steroid medications, often beneficial in reversing a transplant rejection, is not covered by many health insurances, and I am presented alternatives by the insurance company that are so weak they hardly penetrate the ocular surface. The insurance company would rather the patient lose their transplant and require a new one than cover the graft saving medication. It makes no sense—not from a patient suffering prospective or a business perspective for that matter. It costs the system more to replace a transplant; it costs society more to replace a failed transplant. The patient cannot see to drive to work, thus cannot work; they cannot see to care for their family or themselves. The disability paperwork flows in. It starts a viscous spiraling down that could have totally been avoided—just listen to the physician.

Ophthalmologists are trained to save vision, prevent blindness, and improve quality of life (people fear loss of eyesight only second to death), yet we're forced to do so within a system where a bottle of eye drops can cost more than a week's worth of groceries. Access to care shouldn't feel like a luxury item. But for many of my patients, especially in rural West Virginia, the barrier isn't the disease—it's the cost of surviving it.

How Hospitals Profit Off the Ordinary

As a physician, I am acutely aware of the financial disparities that exist within the modern healthcare system, particularly how hospitals and large medical institutions profit disproportionately from both patients and doctors. A personal experience with a close family member brought this issue into sharp focus, leaving me both astonished and deeply concerned about the exploitation taking place within hospital-owned outpatient clinics. Knowing that my family member was at risk for developing glaucoma, I referred them to the Cleveland Clinic Eye Institute's Department of Glaucoma Services. As a physician, I understand that doctors should not be directly involved in the medical or surgical management of their immediate family members, as emotions can cloud clinical judgment. Given that my family member lived in Cleveland, I entrusted their care to the Cleveland Clinic, expecting a standard ophthalmologic evaluation. They attended their appointment at a Cleveland Clinic-affiliated outpatient clinic—not inside a hospital but rather in a standalone medical office building. The visit itself was routine: a comprehensive eye examination, analysis of the optic nerve, and a visual field test—precisely the same evaluation I would have performed in my own clinic using the same equipment and protocols. After a brief consultation with the ophthalmologist, my family member was diagnosed as a glaucoma suspect and was prescribed a nightly eye drop.

What followed was shocking. My family member received a bill in the mail for the visit, totaling $2,781.00—an amount that was 10 times higher than what I would have received for the exact same services in my private practice—approximately $250-$300. And yes, my family member had "good" health insurance. As a fellow sub-specialist, my training and qualifications mirrored those of the doctor who performed the exam at Cleveland Clinic, yet the institution was able to bill—and receive—a dramatically higher reimbursement for identical services. My family member called and sent letters to The Cleveland Clinic, their health insurance company, Aetna, and the State of Ohio's Insurance

Commissioner, all of whom told him the hospital's billing system was allowed.

Where did that extra money go? Certainly not to the doctor who provided the care. Instead, it was funneled into the hospital system, which is legally permitted to bill at hospital-based reimbursement rates, even for visits conducted in outpatient office buildings that are not hospitals. Because Cleveland Clinic owns the outpatient clinic, it is classified as a hospital-affiliated facility. Thus, the same eye exam was billed as if my family member had undergone surgery within a hospital setting despite never setting foot inside an operating room.

This practice is not unique to Cleveland Clinic—it occurs hundreds to thousands of times a day, every single day, across hospital-owned outpatient clinics nationwide. Why do you think hospitals are buying up doctor's outpatient practices across the country at alarming rates? Consider the numbers: An ophthalmologist typically sees 40 to 50 patients per day. Multiply one inflated bill by 40 or 50 patients, and suddenly, a single hospital-employed doctor is generating an astronomical amount of daily revenue for the institution: essentially half of that doctor's annual salary in one day. Scale that across thousands of physicians working within a single hospital system, and then thousands of physicians working in hospital systems all over the country, and the financial picture becomes staggering.

This is a large part of where our healthcare dollars are going (among other places such as executive and administrative salaries as discussed). Hospitals and insurance companies are profiting massively at the expense of both patients and physicians. Meanwhile, the doctors providing the care receive only a minute fraction of the billed amount. Yet when the topic of physician salaries arises, doctors, not the billion-dollar institutions, are labeled as greedy.

More concerning is that patients struggle to afford the care they need to get well. They struggle to afford the necessary medications and procedures. They are kept in the dark with respect to options that can address the root cause of their issues; treatments that can make them well are not covered by their health insurance companies. It would provide no financial benefit to the corporations that profit from keeping patients sick—the pharmaceutical companies, the insurance companies, and the healthcare organizations, hospitals and the like.

I again assert that physicians have become voluntary slaves to a hospital-centric financial model that disproportionately rewards administrative executives and corporate interests rather than those who deliver patient care. Patients, too, suffer under this model as they are required to pay exorbitant costs to meet insurance deductibles before coverage kicks in, only to still owe a percentage of the bill thereafter.

Even more troubling is that most patients do not realize they are being charged excessive hospital-based rates when they visit large academic hospital systems. They assume they are simply receiving standard outpatient care, when in reality, they are being billed as if they had undergone hospital-based procedures. Awareness is crucial. Patients must understand the financial implications of seeking care at hospital-affiliated outpatient clinics and should consider whether seeing a private-practice physician for the same services would be more cost-effective.

This is the reality of our healthcare system—where hospitals and insurers legally exploit both doctors and patients for financial gain, while those who dedicate their lives to patient care receive insufficient compensation for their expertise and time, and patients cannot afford care. It is an unsustainable and morally bankrupt system that must change.

The Illusion of Prestige: The Unseen Costs of Specialization and Academic Medicine

Following residency, doctors have a choice. They can enter practice in their specialty, or they can choose to pursue additional training through a fellowship, where they sub-specialize in a highly specific area of medicine. This means another application process, more interviews, more match fees, and, of course, another year (or more) of grueling training at the same abysmal pay rate as residency.

When a doctor decides to pursue fellowship training, it means they have chosen to sub-specialize within their field to develop an advanced level of expertise in a specific area. For example, when I completed my residency in ophthalmology, I was trained as a comprehensive ophthalmologist, meaning I had received broad education and experience in all aspects of eye care. However, to become highly specialized in a particular area, I chose to undergo an additional year of fellowship training in corneal transplantation and advanced cataract surgery. This extra training, known as a fellowship, is conducted under the guidance of a fellowship mentor who has extensive expertise in that sub-specialty. Once a doctor completes a fellowship, they are no longer considered a generalist within their field but rather a sub-specialist with highly refined skills in a specific niche of their specialty. In my case, this means I am recognized as a corneal transplant specialist within ophthalmology. Other ophthalmologists may choose to specialize further in retina, glaucoma, oculoplastics, or other advanced areas of eye care. Fellowship programs exist across many medical specialties, allowing physicians to super-specialize in their field beyond the general training received in residency.

Following fellowship (or after residency for those who do not pursue a fellowship), a doctor must become board-certified in their specialty. Board certification is granted by the governing board of the doctor's respective specialty and serves as an official validation that the physician possesses the knowledge, skills, and expertise required to practice competently. To obtain board certification, doctors must pass a series of rigorous examinations, typically beginning with a comprehensive multiple-choice test assessing their theoretical knowledge of their field. If they pass this written exam, they must then undergo an oral examination, which is an intense and demanding test of their clinical reasoning and decision-making.

These oral board exams are known for being particularly grueling and high stakes. They are often administered over multiple days in designated central locations across the U.S., such as Chicago or Washington, D.C. During the examination, the doctor moves between different rooms, each staffed by a panel of expert examiners who present complex patient cases and clinical scenarios. The doctor must verbally explain their diagnostic reasoning, management approach, and treatment plan for each case. In ophthalmology, for example, candidates are questioned on various eye diseases, surgical interventions, and emergency cases, and they must articulate their approach in real time under significant pressure. Once the oral exams are completed, doctors must wait several weeks to receive their results. Those who pass receive board certification, an achievement that carries professional prestige and signifies competency within their specialty. Those who fail must retake the exam six months later, adding further financial and emotional burden to the process.

However, obtaining board certification is only the beginning—maintaining board certification is an ongoing commitment that lasts throughout a physician's career. Board-certified doctors must regularly renew their certification, which involves fulfilling a set of continuing medical education (CME) requirements. These include reading and analyzing medical journal articles, completing self-assessment questions and case-based learning modules, attending accredited medical conferences and lectures, and taking periodic multiple-choice recertification exams. This process, known as Maintenance of Certification (MOC), ensures that physicians remain up to date with advancements in medicine and emerging clinical guidelines. While lifelong learning is essential in medicine due to the rapid evolution of technology and treatment protocols, the financial cost of maintaining certification is substantial. Doctors must pay for CME courses, journal subscriptions, board exam fees, and recertification assessments, all of which add an ongoing expense to their profession.

Given the ever-changing landscape of medicine, there is no endpoint to a physician's education. Good doctors remain lifelong learners, continually refining their knowledge and adapting to new research, technologies, and best practices. Unlike many professions where formal education ends after a degree is earned, a physician's training never truly stops. In some states, medical boards even require board certification for physicians to maintain their medical license (*state-specific policies should be verified*). This continuous cycle of education, examination, and certification renewal is essential for ensuring patient safety and high standards of care. However, it also underscores the relentless demands placed on physicians, both intellectually and financially, throughout their careers.

My Choice of Sub-specialty

For me, the choice was clear. I wanted to specialize in cornea transplantation and complex cataract surgery, a decision that meant another year of intense training. I applied to seven fellowship programs, hoping to secure a spot at the prestigious Cincinnati Eye Institute, where the leading expert in cornea transplantation—who was and still is considered one of the best in the world—was training fellows. I was fortunate enough to land that coveted spot. Fellowship was even more grueling than residency, not because the hours were longer, but because the expectations were higher. By this point, I was expected to function independently, yet I was also being taught advanced techniques and procedures that would set me apart in my field. I treated patients from all over the world, patients who traveled thousands of miles just to see my mentor. On our busiest clinic days, we saw nearly 90 patients. On surgical days, we operated on 20 to 30 patients—twice a week.

Fellowship also came with the expectation of research. While publishing in peer-reviewed journals is encouraged in residency, in fellowship, it is mandatory. I collected data, analyzed outcomes, and contributed to the growing body of literature in ophthalmology. By the time I finished my training, there wasn't a single corneal condition I hadn't seen. I could walk into any exam room, take one look at an eye, and instantly know what was wrong and how to treat it. My surgical skills were honed, my instincts sharpened. I had become the kind of surgeon patients trusted, and just as importantly, the kind my mentors trusted with their own patients. Surgical training follows an adage: "See one, do one, teach one." It's a terrifying concept when you really think about it—watch a procedure once, then be expected to perform it yourself. But that's how surgeons are trained. We are required to absorb every detail, to commit procedures to memory, to form a precise mental image so that when it's our turn, we can execute flawlessly. Some surgeons have natural ability. Some do not. There is no test to determine surgical competence when entering a residency or fellowship program. Those without surgical skill are quickly identified. In fellowship, if you aren't trusted with your attending's patients, you simply won't operate. I wasn't one of those people. My hands were good. My instincts were sharp. I excelled in surgery, and my mentors recognized that. But surgical skill isn't the only thing that matters. A surgeon must also be trustworthy, honest, and reliable. It doesn't take long for an attending to determine if a trainee possesses these qualities. As an attending myself later in my career, I could identify in minutes which residents had "it" and which ones didn't. It's also a skill that extends into my position as an employer; I can identify immediately which team members will excel and which will eventually fail.

From Fellowship to Financial Free Fall

Fellowship ends, and the real world begins. Some doctors go into academic medicine, working for universities where they teach residents and care for patients. Others enter private practice, either by joining an existing group or attempting the increasingly rare feat of opening a solo practice. Very few doctors go straight into solo practice. Medical school and residency offer no business training, no guidance on how to manage a practice, no education on contracts, finances, or reimbursement structures. Those who successfully start their own practice usually have an entrepreneurial background or a family mentor who has taught them the ropes. They also need funding—something a young doctor, deeply in debt, simply doesn't have.

Those who choose academic medicine do so knowing they will be paid significantly less than their counterparts in private practice. By the time a physician enters the workforce with a degree that has taken 12 to 13 years post-high school to earn, they are often making less than a pharmaceutical sales rep. A primary care physician might start at $125,000 per year, a surgeon at $175,000—still lower than what some sales reps in the medical industry take home. And let's not forget the looming student loan payments that start immediately upon entering practice, the disability insurance premiums paid monthly, the malpractice insurance premiums, the continuing education fees, licensing fees, and so on.

The irony of academic medicine is that within the physician community, those who stay in academia are viewed as altruistic, committed to research and patient care. Meanwhile, those who enter private practice are often labeled as "money-driven," as if a doctor wanting to be financially secure is somehow unethical. The very profession that demands a decade of training and hundreds of thousands in educational debt has stigmatized the idea of doctors making money. But here's the truth: Academic medicine is a business, just like anything else. As previously discussed, the doctors working in these institutions are not the ones profiting. The institutions themselves receive NIH grants, research contracts, and clinical revenue from patient care, not to mention funding from state governments, local governments, and private donors. In 2021, state and local governments in the United States allocated approximately $377 billion to health and hospital services, representing 10% of their direct general expenditures. This allocation made health and hospital services the third-largest expenditure category for these governments, following public welfare and education.

The money flows into academic institutions in staggering amounts, yet little of it reaches the doctors who make the system function. Physicians in academic medicine are nothing more than cogs in a wheel. They fail to see that without them, the system collapses. Doctors are not trained in business. Most of us sign contracts blindly, trusting institutions that do not have our best interests at heart. Even when we hire attorneys, they are often handpicked by the very organizations about to exploit us. We enter medicine to help people. Instead, we become pawns in a system designed to keep us powerless. Instead of recognizing our own power, doctors show up, see patients, and go home, the same way they have been conditioned to function since the first day of medical school. Doctors do not unite. We do not form unions. We do not demand higher pay, better benefits, or reasonable work hours. We do not demand business education in medical school. Instead, we remain stuck in competition with one another, fighting to be the best, measuring our worth by publications, research, and surgical volume rather than by the value we bring to the system.

Meanwhile, the system watches silently, reaping immense profits while physicians bear the weight of its failures.

Reid: The Caregiver

By that point, I was doing everything.

I was running my own ophthalmology practice. I was raising two little boys, just six and eight. And I was taking care of Reid—cooking for him, managing his appointments, researching new therapies, tracking every lab, every scan, every medication. I became his full-time caregiver, driver, advocate, and unofficial hospice provider. He had moved in with me by then. And still, I went to work every day.

There was no pause button. No sabbatical. No "stepping away." Just the constant weight of doing everything for everyone. And I would do it again in a heartbeat—because I loved him. Because he trusted me. Because I knew the system wouldn't catch him if I didn't.

But it was breaking me.

Reid's treatments weren't working. His oncologists had already said they wouldn't. After the standard therapies failed, they placed him in a clinical trial I knew was a long shot. I read the data. I'd seen the outcomes. I knew what "compassionate use" really meant: We don't know what else to do. Still, we hoped. We always hoped.

But soon after the trial began, his decline was sharp. Fast. He lost weight. Lost energy. The sparkle in his eyes dimmed—not because he was afraid, but because he knew time was closing in. And there was nothing left in the system they hadn't already tried.

I remember putting my kids to bed, quietly closing their door, and then walking across the hall to check Reid's oxygen. Sitting beside his bed, praying his lungs would hold through the night. Some days I'd come home from surgery and walk right into caretaker mode, not even taking off my scrubs. I was stitching eyes by day, and a life together by night. I was washing blood out of sheets and blankets and carpets. I was lying in my bed at night listening for him, hoping he would stop coughing, but scared when he did, that he may be dead.

The medical system had given up on him. But I couldn't. I wasn't ready.

And the truth was, I didn't just feel helpless as his advocate. I felt ashamed as a physician. I couldn't save him. The very tools I had trained my whole life to master—medications, diagnostics, consults—they had all failed him. And I was supposed to be the one person in the world who could make a difference.

But nothing worked. And I was drowning beneath the weight of everything and everyone.

Still, he never once complained. Not about the pain. Not about the doctors. Not even about the dying. He just kept saying, "Thank you for everything you're doing."

It was the system that failed him. Not me.

But it didn't feel that way.

Chapter 7

Not Built for Us: The Hidden Barriers in Medicine

Medicine has long been structured around a traditional male workforce, where doctors were historically expected to prioritize their careers above all else. The system was designed for men with stay-at-home spouses, shaping everything from work schedules to leadership structures and financial incentives. While progress has been made, significant barriers persist for women and underrepresented minorities in medicine. Discrimination, though often subtle, remains a real and persistent issue, affecting career advancement and opportunities. Women now comprise over 50% of U.S. medical school students, yet they remain underrepresented in leadership positions. Despite reaching parity in medical school admissions, only 36% of practicing physicians are women. Leadership gaps are even more pronounced, with less than 18% of hospital CEOs and medical school deans being women. The gender pay gap further reflects this disparity—women physicians earn, on average, 25% less than their male counterparts even when adjusting for specialty and hours worked. Pregnancy and motherhood are often viewed as career liabilities rather than milestones, contributing to higher burnout rates among women doctors.

In a landmark victory for women in medicine, a former UCLA physician was recently awarded $1.4 million after successfully suing the university for gender discrimination and retaliation. Dr. Lauren Pinter-

Brown, a highly respected oncologist and researcher, had spent nearly a decade raising concerns about gender inequity and institutional bias at the David Geffen School of Medicine. Her lawsuit exposed a culture where female physicians, even those in senior positions, were regularly undermined, dismissed, or penalized for speaking up.

Dr. Pinter-Brown's experience was all too familiar to many female physicians across the country. Despite her credentials and accomplishments, she reported being isolated, stripped of leadership duties, and publicly humiliated in professional settings. She was accused of "not being a team player" after advocating for herself and her female colleagues. The final blow came when her professional reputation was called into question without due process—prompting her to file a formal lawsuit.

After years of litigation, a jury unanimously sided with her, awarding both compensatory and punitive damages. The case sent a powerful message: The medical profession, despite its prestige, is not immune to the systemic gender bias that pervades so many institutions. And more importantly, women physicians do not have to remain silent about the injustices they face.

Dr. Pinter-Brown's courage not only affirmed her own worth but also lit a torch for the many women who have been silenced by fear of retaliation or reputational harm. Her story is a reminder that equity in medicine will only be achieved when the profession begins to value the voices of all its members equally—and when institutions are held accountable for the harm they allow or perpetuate.

Medicine Wasn't Built for Mothers

As a female physician, my journey through medicine has been filled with challenges that extend far beyond patient care. In academic medicine, I was bypassed for leadership roles that I had earned. In private practice, I endured workplace harassment during my pregnancy that led to severe stress and resignation.

Gender inequality and systemic biases remain deeply ingrained in the profession, shaping experiences in ways that are both subtle and overt. These disparities have shaped my career, forcing me to make difficult decisions that my male colleagues have rarely had to face. I recall my own pregnancies as a practicing physician at the ages of 34 and 36. It was simply expected, without question or discussion, that I would continue working until the day of my delivery.

There were no conversations about accommodations or adjusted work hours—surgery days then could seem endless—despite the physical toll of pregnancy. At the time of my first pregnancy, I was in academic medicine, and during my second, I was in private practice. My experience in private practice was particularly harrowing. Workplace harassment became so severe that I was placed under intense stress in the final months of pregnancy, leading to multiple hospital visits for Braxton Hicks contractions. Had I not made the difficult decision to resign from my position, my baby could have been born six weeks prematurely.

Resigning from that role meant walking away from financial stability with no new position lined up. Fortunately, I had enough money to sustain myself for the year, during which I focused on caring for my son and seeking a new job. Yet this decision has followed me ever since. On every job application and medical license renewal, I have had to explain the gap in my employment. When I list "parental leave" as the reason, I am met with scrutiny—why did I take so much time off?

Male physicians who take extended time for fellowships, research, or administrative roles are rarely questioned this way. When I did return to work in a new group private practice, I was quickly reminded of the double standard that women in medicine face. On my very first day back performing corneal transplants, the senior cornea surgeon in the practice entered my operating room uninvited, stood over my shoulder, and watched me work. His presence was not out of support or curiosity—he openly stated that because I had been out on leave, he needed to observe my ability. His assumption was clear: My surgical skills had deteriorated during my time away despite the fact that performing corneal transplants is second nature to me—I could perform them in my sleep. Had I been a male surgeon returning from an extended leave for a research sabbatical or administrative role, no such observation or doubt would have been placed on me.

The gender-based discrimination I experienced was not limited to motherhood. Throughout my career, I have faced countless instances of harassment, exclusion, and gender disparity. I often wonder if racial bias played a role as well. While I am Caucasian, I have curly hair and a darker complexion, leading to frequent assumptions in the African American, Puerto Rican, and Hispanic communities that I am of mixed race. This perception may have compounded the bias I encountered in certain professional settings.

One of my earliest experiences with severe gender discrimination occurred during my ophthalmology residency. Six months into my first year, I suffered a devastating house fire that destroyed nearly everything I owned. Though the structural framework of my home remained intact, the interior required a complete rebuild, and I lost all my possessions. I was left without clothing, without a coat, and without the means to replace my professional wardrobe overnight. My sister and mom and dad helped as best they could—my sister, who was several sizes smaller than me at the time, gave me clothes to wear, and my parents took me shopping for essentials, including a winter coat. Instead of receiving support from my residency program, I was called into my program director's office and told that she was aware of the fire but that I should consider buying turtlenecks to wear to work. In that moment, my reality became clear—there was no space for compassion or understanding in this profession. I was expected to simply endure my hardships without complaint, to perform at the same level as everyone else despite suffering a personal crisis. My male colleagues, many of whom had never faced such scrutiny, never received commentary on their attire or personal circumstances.

Dr. Shah reflects on her own difficulties as a mother and woman in medicine. Her decision to leave, as discussed in the chapter on burnout, wasn't just about burnout—it was about boundaries. As a mother and physician, Dr. Shah found herself navigating a system that was never designed with women in mind. The structural rigidity of traditional medicine left little room for caregiving responsibilities—and even less for setting limits without judgment.

"Medicine is still structured for men," says Dr. Shah. "I couldn't attend 7:00 a.m. meetings or work past 3:30 p.m. regularly—I had kids. Those 7:00 a.m. meetings were filled with males—they didn't understand. At Cleveland Clinic, part-time for women physicians meant 32 hours, and we were still expected to keep up. I was seen as less committed just for needing balance." She adds, "I had to enforce boundaries no one else was enforcing. And when you say no, especially as a woman, you're viewed as difficult."

Beauty Bias

In professional environments, women who are perceived as attractive often face unique challenges and biases. Personally, I have encountered situations where my body shape and size have led to perceptions of inappropriate dress despite adhering to standard professional attire. This underscores a broader issue where societal standards and individual perceptions intersect, leading to unfair judgments based on appearance.

Research indicates that attractive women may be subjected to negative stereotypes, including perceptions of reduced competence and trustworthiness. A study published in the *Journal of Management* found that attractive women were often deemed less truthful and more deserving of termination compared to their peers . Additionally, the "beauty is beastly" effect suggests that in certain professional contexts, particularly those traditionally dominated by men, physical attractiveness can be a hindrance for women, leading to assumptions of lesser capability.

The concept of "beauty bias" or "pretty privilege" further complicates this dynamic. While attractive individuals might receive certain societal advantages, these benefits are often accompanied by increased scrutiny and higher expectations. For instance, attractive women may be perceived as using their looks to advance professionally, leading to feelings of jealousy and fear among colleagues . This bias can result in a paradox where beauty becomes both an asset and a liability in professional settings.

Moreover, dress code policies in workplaces can disproportionately impact women, especially those with certain body types. Women often navigate a fine line between appearing too plain and being perceived as overly provocative. This balancing act can lead to unwarranted criticisms and assumptions about professionalism based solely on appearance.

Beauty bias is deeply ingrained in medicine, where female physicians who are perceived as attractive often face the assumption that they are nurses, assistants, or incapable of intellectual rigor. Patients and even male colleagues may subconsciously equate appearance with incompetence, undermining our authority before we've spoken a word. Addressing these biases requires a conscious effort to challenge societal stereotypes and promote a more inclusive understanding of professionalism that values competence over appearance.

In my last private practice group, I experienced one of the most humiliating moments of my career. A senior male physician in the group—one who had attempted to use his power and influence over me—bullied me, tarnished my name, and ensured that his reputation remained intact while mine suffered. Even after I left and started my own practice, my name continued to be dragged through professional circles. In line with the "beauty bias," the female staff members in that practice referred to me in the community as someone who dressed inappropriately, further attempting to discredit my professionalism. Meanwhile, I was laughed at and labeled as an "alpha female"—a derogatory term used to describe women who assert themselves in a field where confidence and leadership are expected traits for men.

In the same practice, I was openly referred to as a bitch—not because of incompetence or wrongdoing, but simply for excelling in my field and refusing to be controlled. In one of the most competitive specialties in medicine, a female surgeon must be assertive, decisive, and technically excellent, yet these same qualities, when displayed by a woman, trigger resentment and an inferiority complex among male colleagues.

The very traits that make a successful surgeon—confidence, precision, leadership, and ambition—are the same traits that cause female surgeons to be criticized, ostracized, and penalized in the workplace.

The reality is this: Women in medicine are held to a different standard. We are expected to prove ourselves repeatedly, and even when we do, we are still questioned, undervalued, and underpaid. Pregnancy is treated as an inconvenience rather than a natural part of life. Maternity leave is scrutinized, while men's extended leaves for research or administrative duties are respected. Harassment and discrimination are systemic issues, yet when we speak out, we are labeled as difficult, ungrateful, or too emotional.

Despite these challenges, I persisted, built my own practice, and thrived—but at what cost? How many women have left medicine entirely due to these same obstacles? How many brilliant female physicians have been denied leadership opportunities, pushed out of their specialties, or have chosen to sacrifice their careers for the well-being of their families?

Until these issues are acknowledged and addressed, the gender disparities in medicine will continue, forcing women to navigate a system that was never designed for them. Medicine's work schedules remain designed for a 1950s family model, assuming that physicians can dedicate 60 to 80 hours per week indefinitely while leaving personal responsibilities to a spouse.

For women, who still bear the majority of household and childcare duties, this structure creates an impossible choice: sacrifice family for career or sacrifice career advancement for family, often resulting in reduced opportunities and lower pay. The stigma surrounding maternity leave persists, with many residency programs lacking formal policies and female physicians fearing career repercussions if they take time off. As a new mother, and an assistant professor in academic medicine, I had no private space to pump breast milk during my workday. I shared an office with my secretary, and the only place I could find any semblance of privacy was a restroom—a humiliating and deeply unsanitary option, yet for five years, it was my only one.

Countless stories like mine exist of pregnant doctors working through complications just to avoid appearing weak or uncommitted to their profession.

Still Paid Less: The Persistent Gender Pay Gap in Healthcare

Even when controlling for factors such as specialty and hours worked, the gender pay gap persists. A 2021 study found that male physicians earn, on average, $100,000 more per year than their female colleagues. Women are also less likely to receive bonuses or leadership opportunities despite having equal qualifications. Leadership in medicine remains a "boys' club," where men are more likely to mentor and promote other men, and women are often held to higher performance standards while facing harsher criticism for demonstrating leadership traits. Women doctors are less likely to be promoted to department chair, medical director, or hospital CEO, and more likely to be overlooked for high-paying sub-specialties.

I learned this the hard way. Early in my career, I stood up for myself in academic medicine. I refused to be undervalued, and for that, I was labeled a troublemaker. As a female surgeon, I was overlooked for promotional opportunities despite being more qualified than my male colleagues. I remember when the head of our cornea and refractive department left for private practice. He was a prominent figure, not just within our institution but in the global ophthalmology community. He had recruited me into the program, and I had earned his trust. I handled his corneal surgical complications. I had believed he valued me as a colleague, but I was just another fellow in his eyes. When he left, he offered me a position as an employee in his new private practice—but on the condition that I would go without a salary. I would be expected to take home whatever I could collect from patient insurance, but not before paying my personal overhead (as if I owned the practice, but I had no ownership and never would) and him and his partners, 40% of my collections first. Even at 35, still earning $200,000 annually in academia, I knew a bad deal when I saw one. I declined and stayed in the institution.

While a better decision than joining my colleague in his practice, my decision to remain at the same academic institution was wrong and did not last long. The refractive and surgical center this man had overseen was left without leadership when he exited. I was the logical choice to step into his role. I had the expertise, the experience, and the proven surgical outcomes. Instead, a glaucoma specialist with no refractive surgery experience was given the position because he was friends with the department chairman. That was the moment I knew I had to leave. When I finally decided to walk away, I had to fight to get the money I had earned. My contract stated that once I generated three times my salary, I was entitled to 40% of my additional collections. I surpassed that easily, even within the slow, bureaucratic billing system of academia. Yet when I requested the money I had rightfully earned, my chairman looked me in the eye and said, "I think I've paid you enough." I had to file a complaint with the Dean of the institution. Thankfully, she was a woman, recently appointed as part of a package deal when her husband was hired as a retina specialist in our department. The previous female retina specialist had left in disgust over the leadership. Six months later, after I had already left, I finally received the money I had worked for.

When Medicine Doesn't Reflect the People It Serves

Beyond gender disparities, medicine remains overwhelmingly white despite the increasingly diverse U.S. population. Only 5% of U.S. doctors are Black, while 6% are Hispanic. Minority students face higher barriers to entering medical school, and minority patients struggle to find doctors who share their background. The cost of medical school— often exceeding $200,000 in debt-disproportionately affects Black and Hispanic students, who are less likely to come from backgrounds with generational wealth. Systemic barriers to medical education include limited access to academic mentorship, MCAT prep courses, and financial resources, all of which contribute to the lack of racial diversity in the profession.

The lack of diversity extends beyond admissions and into academic medicine and leadership. The majority of medical school faculty remain white men, and minority physicians often struggle to find mentors who understand their unique challenges. Bias in residency selection still favors traditional majority—white networks and implicit discrimination affects hiring and promotion decisions. Minority physicians report higher rates of discrimination from patients, colleagues, and hospital staff, with Black and Hispanic female doctors facing compounded biases due to both gender and racial discrimination.

The lack of diversity in medicine has real consequences for patient care. Studies show that Black patients have better health outcomes when treated by Black doctors, and Hispanic patients report higher trust in healthcare providers who share their background. Minority communities are less likely to seek medical care when they do not see themselves represented in the profession.

Similarly, when women are excluded from leadership roles, workplace policies fail to accommodate the realities of motherhood, contributing to higher burnout rates and physician attrition. The healthcare system loses the benefits of diverse leadership, which could improve decision-making and patient outcomes.

Addressing these disparities requires systemic reform at multiple levels. Medical schools and residency programs must increase diversity in admissions, offer financial assistance for underrepresented students, and implement formal maternity leave policies. Hospitals must work to close the gender pay gap, track salary discrepancies, and ensure fair promotions. Leadership opportunities for women and minorities must be expanded to break the cycle of exclusion that has persisted for decades.

For individual physicians, advocacy is key. Women and minority doctors must push for leadership roles, demand fair pay, and support organizations that promote diversity in medicine. Mentorship and sponsorship programs should be expanded to help underrepresented physicians navigate institutional bias and advance in their careers. Medicine must evolve to reflect the diverse population it serves. Doctors should never have to choose between their careers and their families, and racial and gender bias should have no place in a profession built on saving lives. The future of medicine must be more inclusive, but this change will not happen automatically. It requires policy shifts, institutional reform, and cultural transformation within the profession. Diversity in medicine doesn't just benefit doctors—it saves lives.

Chapter 8

The Pressure of Patients on Doctors: The Duality of the Doctor-Patient Relationship

Most patients are kind. They are grateful, appreciative, and respectful of their doctors. I have patients who bring me gifts around the holidays, boxes of sweets, handmade goods, thank-you cards, and flowers. Patient referrals are the best referrals. When a patient tells me they have recommended me to a friend or family member, I tell them how much that means to me, because it is personal. It's not another doctor saying, "Go see this specialist." It is someone who has been in my care, who has trusted me with their health, and who has found that experience so valuable that they want someone they love to experience it, too.

I enjoy my patients. I love getting to know them, hearing their stories, and playing a part in their health and healing. But as much as I love them, I have also felt the weight of their expectations, the pressure that can be crushing, the demand that can push me beyond my own human limits.

Being a doctor is a lot like being a mother. When a mother has a sick child, she devotes all her time and energy to making sure that child is okay. A mother doesn't sleep if her child is up crying. She neglects her own meals, her own needs, her own health, because all that matters in that moment is making sure her child recovers. The mother will wait on that child hand and foot, comforting them, making sure they are warm, making sure they have what they need. She will put aside her own exhaustion, her own headache, her own aches and pains, because her child is depending on her.

Doctors live this experience, except instead of caring for one sick child, we are responsible for thousands. Thousands of patients who rely on us, who come to us for answers, who expect us to be there when they need us. And if we fumble, if we make one human error, if we miss a single step, we risk losing everything. A mother who makes a mistake while caring for her sick child is forgiven. A doctor who makes a mistake can lose their license, their reputation, and their career.

Most patients are genuine, but the system is set up in such a way that some see their doctors as easy targets for blame, for frustration, for lawsuits and monetary gain. The healthcare system is designed to protect patients above all else, which means doctors often find themselves unprotected, vulnerable, and subject to scrutiny that has little to do with their actual performance or medical judgment.

In many states, a patient can file a grievance against a doctor with the medical board, and the board is required to investigate, regardless of whether the claim has merit. The mere accusation is enough to set an entire process into motion, forcing a doctor to spend months defending themselves, sometimes hiring attorneys, always under the stress of knowing that no matter how well they documented their decisions, no matter how ethically or carefully they practiced, their career is on the line.

I once endured an excruciating six-month battle with my state medical board after a patient filed a complaint against me. He had a blind, painful eye and had consulted me for a cornea transplant. I declined to perform the surgery, not because I didn't want to help him, but because it was unethical to transplant a cornea into an eye with no potential for vision. That cornea could have gone to someone else, someone who had a chance to see again. I offered him alternative treatments for pain relief. I explained the reasoning behind my decision. I documented everything. I even offered to send him for a second opinion, which he refused.

Still, he filed a grievance against me, claiming I had neglected to treat his pain. It took me half a year and the cost of a lawyer to clear my name, even though my documentation showed I had gone above and beyond to help him. He was frustrated with his situation, and I became his target.

Not long after that, I had another patient file a complaint. He had developed an infection inside the eye after an intraocular surgery and was at high risk of complications due to his poor health and diabetes. I did exactly what the standard of care required—I referred him to a retina specialist for treatment. He received an injection, his infection cleared, and he regained his full sight.

Yet he still filed a complaint, not because of his outcome, but because I had not personally called to check on him after transferring his care. I had been receiving updates from his treating doctor, but I had not personally picked up the phone. That was enough to put me through another six months of legal headaches. He was not wrong. I could have called him. I did not intentionally neglect to call him. I am sure I was busy seeing other patients, running a business, being a mom, and it did not cross my mind. I cared about him and was so happy for his positive outcome. Does my lack of a phone call really necessitate a medical board investigation? I would have rather he called me and just asked why I had not personally checked on him.

Some states have better systems in place. They screen complaints to determine if they warrant a full investigation. But in my state, every complaint moves forward, no matter how frivolous. It doesn't matter if the doctor acted with care, if the outcome was good, or if the complaint is rooted in emotion rather than negligence. The process itself is punishment enough.

On top of the legal vulnerability doctors face, patients also expect us to always be available. Taking a vacation is difficult. Even when I plan my time off a year in advance, I still return to patients who are surprised or even irritated that I was unavailable. "I tried to call, but you were on vacation," they'll say, with a tone that suggests I shouldn't have been. "Why do you need a vacation? Aren't doctors supposed to be available?"

Patients have yelled at my staff for my absence. They have been angry when I was unavailable for one week out of an entire year. They forget that I, too, am human.

If my child is sick, or if I am sick, it is the end of the world to cancel a patient's appointment. In 20 years of practice, I can count on one hand the number of times I have called in sick. I can only recall three times that I physically could not come to work, and each of those times, I was so sick I could barely stand. I have gone to work with migraines, body aches, extreme fatigue. I have seen patients while feeling like I would collapse. Doctors are trained to push through, to keep going, to sacrifice themselves for the sake of others.

I have left my sick child with a relative so I could go take care of someone else. I have ignored my own exhaustion, my own pain, because that is what is expected of me. And still, there are those who believe doctors are overpaid, greedy, only in it for the money.

I once had a patient's husband look me in the eye after I came into the room 30 minutes late. This was when Reid was in the hospital, dying. The night before this, he had an episode of bleeding in his lungs that could not be stopped. I had spent the night in the hospital with him, knowing he was dying, holding his hand through his final hours.

That morning, I left him for a short time to see the few patients who were waiting for me in clinic. When I apologized to this man for my delay, when I explained to him that my brother was dying, he looked at me and said, "I don't care about that. My wife has an appointment, and it's your job to see her."

I didn't have the energy to fight with him. I just cried, right there, right then. I saw his wife and let them go. I fired them from my care after that, because I could not look at them again.

I have had patients scream at me in the hallway that I make too much money. I have had patients accuse me of ordering unnecessary tests just for financial gain, not realizing that I do not receive a cent from the labs I order. There is this strange, persistent belief that doctors are making too much money, that we are somehow undeserving of financial success despite the sacrifices we have made, the years of training, the debt, the long hours, the legal risks, and the personal toll this career takes.

Where does this belief come from? Why are we not outraged at the millions spent on athletes, hedge fund managers, and healthcare executives, yet we resent the idea of a physician being well compensated? Why do we undervalue the very people responsible for keeping us alive?

Dr. Shah has experienced patient abuse in a traumatic and personal way. While building her integrative medicine clinic, she was physically assaulted by a patient who threw her to the ground by her ponytail. "She was a therapist," Shah says. "Not someone off the street. But I was traumatized. I sued for workers' compensation and never went back to that clinic. I had PTSD for months. There are no protections in place for us." She notes how common it is for physicians—especially women—to tolerate abuse, and how systems rarely intervene until it's too late.

The psychological wounds in medicine often go unseen. Dr. Shah's experience with workplace assault left her with post-traumatic stress disorder, but the bigger issue, she says, was how normalized it was to suffer in silence. "We're expected to take it. If you say something, you're a liability. So, you internalize it—and it eats at you."

Misdirected Frustration

Patients are growing increasingly frustrated with the rising costs of healthcare and the barriers preventing them from accessing the care they need. Insurance premiums, deductibles, denials, long wait times, and out-of-pocket expenses have made even basic healthcare feel inaccessible to many Americans. But rather than directing their anger toward the bureaucratic systems, insurance conglomerates, and corporate healthcare structures responsible for these limitations, that frustration is often tragically misdirected, aimed instead at the doctors themselves. One of the most shocking examples of this misplaced rage came in early 2024, when a Utah man fatally shot Dr. Marc Harrison, the former CEO of Intermountain Healthcare. The man, a patient with long-standing grievances about the healthcare system, claimed in his online posts that he had been mistreated, dismissed, and financially ruined by medical expenses. Though Dr. Harrison was no longer serving as CEO at the time of his death, he became the symbolic target of a man's bottled-up rage—rage that had been simmering within a system that routinely fails both patients and providers. What this tragedy highlights is the growing disconnect between the public and the profession of medicine. Many patients no longer see physicians as allies but as gatekeepers to a system that appears indifferent to their suffering. What they don't realize is that most physicians are equally trapped, working within a profit-driven model that often restricts their ability to provide the care they were trained to give. Doctors are fighting to navigate a maze of administrative tasks, insurance denials, and limited resources, all while trying to maintain empathy and connection in an increasingly hostile environment.

The Doctor as a Clerk

Beyond mistrust and violence, modern doctors now face another quiet assault—death by paperwork. As our authority wanes, our time is consumed not by patients, but by administrative tasks that devalue our expertise and erode our time. It is now commonplace that when a doctor writes a prescription for a patient, that prescription is returned by the pharmacy stating the "insurance" requires an alternative.

Doctors and nurses spend endless unreimbursed hours working on the completion of prior authorizations for medications and medical visits and procedures as insurance companies force us to find the cheapest solution to the patient's problem as opposed to the doctor's recommendation. Patients do not understand the hurdle and call the doctor's office repeatedly, frustrated with the physician, not understanding the battle required to get them what they need.

In no other professional environment is an individual, with as much training as a doctor, required to be subservient to individuals with not near the training and expertise and required to work endless hours without being compensated; in no other profession is a professional required to answer phone calls and emails without being compensated, or risk a malpractice charge due to negligence. Every day, I receive medical records requests from health insurance companies reviewing my documented plans of action in how I have chosen to treat my patients. To assimilate 50 or more patient records and submit them in entirety to a health insurance company for review is not only humiliating but also a time-consuming task that sometimes takes hours to complete; and this must be done without compensation and is requested on a routine basis. I feel like I am submitting an assignment to a teacher for a grade. Do I get an "A" or an "F?" I pay my staff to complete this work for the health insurance company so that the patient may have their visit covered.

This example amplifies the fact that the working conditions of doctors have worsened significantly over the years. In the past, doctors had full control over their practices. They determined their own schedules, set fair fees for their work, and worked within a system that did not involve insurance interference. Today, most doctors are overworked and underpaid for the hours they put in. Long gone are the days of professional autonomy; now, doctors must navigate a sea of bureaucracy, mountains of electronic paperwork, and administrative burdens that detract from patient care. Many physicians find themselves burned out, disillusioned, and questioning whether they can sustain a career in medicine under such conditions.

Why More Doctors Are Leaving Medicine

With all the sacrifice, training, and investment that goes into becoming a physician, one might assume that once doctors finally finish residency and enter practice, they are happy and fulfilled. Unfortunately, more physicians than ever are walking away from medicine entirely or searching for alternative careers. What's driving this exodus? It's not just the long hours or the stress of the job—doctors have always worked hard. The difference now is that the entire healthcare system is broken, and physicians have less autonomy, less time with patients, and more bureaucratic burdens than ever before. Medicine is no longer driven by doctors. It is driven by hospital administrators, insurance companies, and government regulations. Doctors are often forced to prioritize billing codes and insurance approvals over patient care. Instead of seeing patients, doctors now spend more than half their time documenting in clunky electronic medical records systems that were designed for billing, not for patient care. Despite all the years of training, physician salaries have not kept up with inflation, while overhead costs (malpractice insurance, licensing fees, EMR systems, etc.) continue to rise. Many doctors, especially in private practice, struggle to remain financially viable. Many doctors are also working in hostile work environments. Healthcare has become increasingly corporate, and many hospitals treat physicians as replaceable employees rather than respected professionals. Many doctors feel disrespected, undervalued, and expendable in their own institutions. The result? More doctors are choosing early retirement, concierge medicine, telemedicine, or completely non-clinical careers. Others are leaving traditional medical practice to pursue coaching, consulting, entrepreneurship, or wellness careers. Some move into hospital administration themselves, attempting to create change from within.

Chapter 9

The Shrinking Role of the Physician

Over the past two decades, a silent transformation has taken place within healthcare—one that is changing not only how care is delivered, but *who* delivers it. Hospitals and health systems, under pressure to cut costs and address staffing shortages, have increasingly turned to nurse practitioners (NPs) and physician assistants (PAs) to fill roles once exclusively held by physicians. While these professionals are an important part of the care team, their rise as physician substitutes raises urgent questions about clinical depth, patient safety, and what may be lost when years of medical training are sidelined in the name of efficiency. This chapter explores the consequences of this shift—and why physicians must not remain silent as their roles are redefined.

Trend of Replacing Physicians with NPs and PAs

The evolving landscape of healthcare delivery has led to a notable trend: hospitals increasingly employing nurse practitioners (NPs) and physician assistants (PAs) in roles traditionally held by physicians. This shift is primarily driven by efforts to reduce operational costs and address physician shortages. However, this practice raises concerns regarding the quality of patient care, given the significant differences in training and clinical experience between these healthcare professionals.

A study analyzing Medicare data revealed that from 2013 to 2019, the proportion of healthcare visits managed by non-physician clinicians, including NPs and PAs, rose from 14% to 26%. This trend is partly attributed to the rapid growth in the number of NPs and PAs entering the workforce. Projections indicate that between 2019 and 2031, the employment of NPs is expected to increase by 46%, and PAs by 28%, while physician employment is anticipated to grow by only 3%.

Financial considerations also play a significant role in this shift. NPs and PAs generally command lower salaries compared to physicians, making them a cost-effective alternative for healthcare facilities aiming to manage expenses without compromising service delivery. However, this substitution raises critical questions about the equivalence of care provided.

Differences in Training and Clinical Experience

The educational and clinical training pathways for physicians, NPs, and PAs differ substantially. Physicians undergo extensive training, including four years of medical school followed by three to seven years of residency, accumulating between 12,000 to 16,000 hours of patient-care experience. In contrast, NPs typically complete a master's or doctoral degree in nursing, with clinical training ranging from 500 to 1,500 hours. PAs earn a master's degree and undertake approximately 2,000 hours of clinical rotations.

These disparities in training and clinical exposure are significant. While NPs and PAs are integral to the healthcare system and provide valuable services, their comparatively limited training may impact their ability to manage complex medical cases independently. This concern is underscored by the American Medical Association's stance that the extensive education and training of physicians are crucial for optimal patient care, especially in emergencies or complicated scenarios.

Implications for Patient Care

The substitution of physicians with NPs and PAs has sparked debate regarding patient safety and care quality. Instances have been reported where inadequate supervision of less experienced practitioners led to adverse patient outcomes. For example, a case in the UK involved a misdiagnosis by a physician associate (a role similar to PAs in the U.S.), resulting in a patient's death and subsequent calls for stricter regulations and oversight. Such incidents highlight the potential risks associated with replacing highly trained physicians with practitioners who have substantially less clinical experience.

When Titles Blur and Lines Cross: The Push for Surgical Privileges Without Surgical Training

Perhaps the most concerning development in this movement to substitute physicians is the growing push by non-physician practitioners—not only NPs and PAs, but also optometrists—to gain surgical privileges traditionally reserved for medical doctors and surgeons. As an ophthalmologist and corneal transplant surgeon, I find this trend deeply alarming.

Optometrists, though valuable in providing vision screenings and managing basic eye care, are not medical doctors. They do not attend medical school, nor do they complete years of surgical residency. And yet in my home state of West Virginia, legislation was recently passed allowing optometrists to perform certain eye surgeries—despite the fact that their training includes zero hours of live human surgical experience under supervision in accredited residency programs.

As of 2025, optometrists in 13 U.S. states are authorized to perform certain in-office laser and minor surgical procedures. These procedures include selective laser trabeculoplasty (SLT), YAG capsulotomy, lesion removal, and specific injections. There are six additional states actively considering similar scope expansions.

This isn't a philosophical disagreement—it's a patient safety issue.

Granting surgical privileges to providers who haven't been trained in the operating room under the high-pressure, high-risk realities of surgery does not serve rural communities—it endangers them. Those who support these policies often argue that expanding optometrists' scope of practice helps increase access to care. But access to substandard or unsafe care is not progress. It is a disservice cloaked as a solution.

In states like West Virginia, where physician shortages are real and healthcare access is often limited by geography and poverty, it may seem tempting to blur professional lines for the sake of convenience. But patients in rural areas deserve the same standard of care as those in urban centers. They deserve physicians trained to handle complications, not providers practicing procedures they were never adequately trained to perform.

As someone who has spent years restoring vision through delicate microsurgery, I know firsthand how much skill, repetition, judgment, and anatomical understanding are required to achieve successful outcomes. The notion that this can be replaced by short courses or simulators is both naive and dangerous.

This isn't about professional competition. It's about protecting the public. When we begin to trade depth of training for convenience and clinical expertise for budgetary efficiency, we are setting a precedent that may be difficult to reverse—and the casualties will not be on paper. They will be real people, with real complications, facing real harm.

Real Consequences: When Lives and Vision Are on the Line

This issue is not theoretical for me. I have personally seen the devastating consequences when surgical decision-making and postoperative management are placed in the hands of individuals who do not have the appropriate training, clinical judgment, or experience.

Patient Case #1: Missed Diagnosis, Irreversible Harm

One of the most sobering cases I've encountered involved a woman who was evaluated for LASIK surgery by a local optometrist. He deemed her a good candidate and coordinated the surgery with a refractive surgeon who traveled in from out of state. This setup—an OD making surgical clearance decisions and a surgeon relying solely on that advice—was the first critical error.

The patient had two absolute contraindications for LASIK: an inherited condition called Fuchs' endothelial dystrophy, a cornea condition that can eventually lead to the need for cornea transplant, and a visually significant cataract. Any corneal surgeon knows that performing LASIK in these conditions is dangerous and reckless. Yet the procedure went forward.

Postoperatively, she developed a severe corneal ulcer, which the optometrist attempted to manage himself. The surgeon had already returned to his home state and was unavailable. By the time she was referred to me, her cornea had perforated, meaning a hole had formed in the center of her eye. I had no choice but to perform an emergent corneal transplant to salvage her vision. She later sued the optometrist, but he had moved out of state to Kentucky, and despite the egregious mismanagement, she was unable to win the case. She lost more than a lawsuit—she lost trust, function, and a piece of herself. She won a lifetime of biannual cornea transplant visits and daily anti-rejection eye drops.

Patient Case #2: Delayed Referral, Permanent Damage

Another recent case involved a man who wore contact lenses and developed a corneal ulcer. He sought care from an optometrist who mismanaged him for weeks without improvement; the optometrist treated him with topical steroid drops, a known contraindication to an active cornea ulcer. By the time the patient reached me, he had a full-thickness fungal ulcer that had invaded the eye. This was not a common infection. It was rare, aggressive, and required immediate action.

He underwent an emergent corneal transplant to save his eye, as well as months of oral anti-fungal agents to avoid retinal involvement. It was a stark example of how dangerous delays in proper care can be, and how even well-meaning providers, when working outside their depth, can cause irreversible harm.

These are not isolated incidents. They are the predictable result of a system that blurs roles and prioritizes cost savings over clinical training. In both cases, earlier involvement by a trained ophthalmologist would have prevented the complications entirely. These stories are burned into my memory, and they are far from unique.

Published Case Study Supporting These Concerns

Delayed Referral of Sight-Threatening Eye Conditions

A large study conducted in the UK found that delays in referral to ophthalmologists by optometrists and general practitioners contributed to worsened outcomes in conditions such as retinal detachment, uveitis, and keratitis. The authors concluded that earlier intervention by ophthalmologists was key to preserving vision.

While integrating nurse practitioners (NPs) and physician assistants (PAs) into healthcare teams is an important step in addressing provider shortages and expanding access to care, it is imperative that we recognize the critical differences in education, clinical experience, and scope of practice between these roles and that of a physician. Collaborative care can absolutely improve outcomes when it is structured around the unique strengths and limits of each professional. But replacing physicians outright, particularly in complex or high-risk medical situations, is a shortcut that risks sacrificing safety for efficiency.

Even more alarming is the growing trend of granting surgical privileges to optometrists, a move that goes beyond collaborative care into dangerous territory. Optometrists, while highly skilled in primary eye care and vision correction, do not undergo medical school or surgical residency training. When they are allowed to perform procedures that require advanced anatomical knowledge and intraoperative judgment, we place patients at unnecessary risk. The recent legislation in West Virginia, which now permits optometrists to perform certain eye surgeries, is not progress—it is a step backward in the standards of medical safety and training.

If we continue down this road—where clinical complexity is handed off to those without the appropriate depth of preparation—we must ask ourselves: What exactly are we optimizing for? Cheaper labor? Shorter wait times? Or true health outcomes?

The answer should always be the same: patient safety, quality care, and the preservation of clinical excellence. Anything less is not innovation. It's abandonment.

Reid: Austria

We were out of options—or so we were told.

Standard treatment had failed. The clinical trial, as I feared, only accelerated his decline. He was losing weight rapidly. His breath was shorter. And yet his spirit? Unchanged. Reid was still Reid. Still cracking jokes. Still thanking nurses. Still showing more grace than most people do in perfect health.

But I knew we couldn't wait any longer. I was done with watching the system throw darts in the dark while pretending they were evidence-based miracles. We needed a new path. A new philosophy. Something that actually made sense.

That's when we found Dr. Ralf Kleef, MD.

A naturopathic oncologist I trusted, Dr. Natalie Winters, mentioned his name to me. She spoke about him like people talk about folklore. A sarcoma specialist in Vienna, Austria. Trained at MD Anderson and Sloan Kettering but no longer part of that world. He had gone a different way. A better way. He was treating patients with protocols no one here dared to try—mistletoe, hyperthermia, low-dose immunotherapy, high-

dose vitamin C, checkpoint inhibitors. Not to suppress the body, but to empower it.

He had documented success. Real cases. Remissions that defied expectation. Young patients with the same diagnosis as Reid—alive, thriving, years later. It felt like someone had cracked open a hidden door I'd been banging on my whole career.

We booked the Skype call with Dr. Kleef. I remember Reid sitting beside me, listening carefully as Dr. Kleef explained his philosophy—not just the science, but the soul behind it. He spoke to Reid like a person, not a protocol. Like someone whose life was still worth fighting for, not just someone biding time. I could see the hope return to Reid's eyes.

It was decided. We would go.

We booked flights. He passed his pulmonary clearance. We gathered paperwork, scans, lab results. We were moving fast, fueled by adrenaline and faith. We were going to Austria. We were going to fight differently.

And for the first time in a long time, I felt like a doctor again. Not a system operator. Not a burned-out technician buried in charting and billing codes. I felt like someone on a mission. Like a healer.

Because Reid wasn't a case. He was my family.

And this time, we weren't asking permission to try.

We were going to reclaim his care—and our hope.

Chapter 10

Functional Medicine: A Paradigm Shift in Patient Care

Functional medicine, often referred to as root-cause medicine, is a radically different approach to healthcare—one that prioritizes identifying and addressing the underlying cause of disease rather than simply treating symptoms with pharmaceuticals. Traditional medical training teaches physicians to diagnose based on symptoms and prescribe medications, often without questioning why the patient developed the condition in the first place. This reactive approach leads to a cascade of prescriptions, where each medication's side effects create new health problems, necessitating even more medications.

Take, for example, hypertension. In conventional medicine, a patient with high blood pressure is prescribed antihypertensive medications, often with little discussion about the lifestyle factors that may be contributing to the condition. While medication can be necessary in acute situations, particularly if a patient is at immediate risk for stroke or heart attack, the long-term goal in functional medicine is to identify and correct the root cause—whether it be chronic inflammation, insulin resistance, stress, poor diet, or mineral deficiencies—rather than permanently relying on medication.

The same concept applies to autoimmune diseases, which affect a large percentage of the population. In traditional medicine, autoimmune conditions are classified based on which part of the body is affected—

rheumatoid arthritis attacks the joints, psoriasis attacks the skin, Sjogren's syndrome affects the lacrimal and salivary glands. However, these conditions all stem from the same underlying dysfunction: an overactive immune system driven by chronic inflammation.

Instead of investigating what triggered the immune dysregulation, conventional medicine's approach is to suppress the immune system using powerful immunosuppressive drugs, leaving patients vulnerable to infections, cancers, and long-term side effects. Functional medicine, in contrast, focuses on identifying the triggers—which can include chronic viral infections (such as Epstein-Barr), mold toxicity, environmental toxins, stress, and gut dysbiosis—and addressing them directly.

In my ophthalmology practice, Bellasee™, I have integrated functional medicine principles into the daily care of my ophthalmology patients. When patients present with chronic corneal fungal infections, I test their urine for mycotoxins, identifying the presence of underlying mold exposure. When patients have ocular autoimmune conditions, I investigate whether chronic viral infections or toxin exposures are driving their disease. Instead of defaulting to immunosuppressive therapy, I work to remove the underlying trigger, allowing the body to heal naturally. Of course, there are cases where pharmaceutical interventions are necessary—but my goal is always to use them temporarily while working toward true resolution of the problem.

At Bellasee™, we have also incorporated IV nutrition therapy, recognizing that micronutrient imbalances play a critical role in eye health and systemic disease. We treat the whole person, not just the eyeball—because the eyes are a direct reflection of what is happening in the body as a whole.

Medical schools must begin incorporating functional medicine into their curriculum. Physicians need to be trained to identify root causes, not just match symptoms with pharmaceuticals. Insurance companies must start covering lab work, nutritional therapies, and alternative treatments that actually help patients heal, rather than only covering medications that perpetuate disease.

Physicians who have awakened to functional medicine are leaving traditional practice and risking everything to do what is right for their patients. Typically, traditionally trained medical doctors only learn of functional medicine when they experience a personal health crisis—or their loved ones do—the same experience that I had. This is unacceptable. We, as physicians and as a society, must advocate for change—not just in how we treat our patients, but in how we train the next generation of doctors.

Make no mistake—there is a place for conventional medicine. Emergency medicine saves lives. Advanced cancer treatments and surgical innovations have transformed modern medicine. But for the millions of patients suffering from chronic conditions like hypertension, diabetes, and autoimmune disease, the current system is failing them. They don't need lifelong medications—they need a path to true healing.

The future of medicine must evolve—not to serve corporate interests, but to serve the patients who trust us with their lives.

Honoring Jennifer's Path

This book has spoken openly about the dangers of substituting physicians with lesser-trained providers in high-stakes medical environments. Those concerns remain valid, particularly when it comes to surgical and complex diagnostic care. But that does not mean all non-physician providers are interchangeable—or that their stories don't matter.

Jennifer Bouchard is a nurse practitioner whose journey is not one of substitution but transformation. After witnessing the failures of conventional oncology during her daughter Hannah's cancer battle, Jennifer stepped beyond the limitations of the system—not to replace doctors, but to redefine what healing can look like. She pursued functional oncology, studied emerging therapies, and built a functional oncology practice grounded in compassion, science, and lived experience.

Her story is not an argument for replacing physicians—it is a testament to what happens when a clinician, regardless of credentials, chooses to rise above the system and create something better. Jennifer is not working outside of her depth; she is working beyond its walls.

This story is not about scope. It's about soul.

And it belongs in these pages.

To Hannah:

In 2019, nurse practitioner Jennifer Bouchard's life changed forever. Her daughter Hannah—only 30 years old and a chiropractor—began to experience sudden jaw and ear pain. The initial diagnosis? TMJ. No one looked further. No red flags were raised. Even as the pain became excruciating, no deeper evaluation was done. What should have been a warning sign of something far more serious was brushed aside.

Jennifer, already working at the Cleveland Clinic Center for Functional Medicine, felt something wasn't right. She pushed for answers. By January 2020, a CT scan revealed positive lymph nodes on both sides of Hannah's neck. Still, there was no clear diagnosis—just frustration and delay. Jennifer, as a mother and as a trained provider, demanded an MRI. What it revealed was devastating: a large mass at the base of Hannah's skull. She had Stage IV nasopharyngeal carcinoma. There was only one relevant study—out of Japan—that Jennifer could even find linking the tumor markers.

Hannah underwent high-dose chemotherapy at Yale in early March of 2020—just one week before the world shut down from COVID. She and Jennifer moved into a condo nearby. Jennifer administered IV therapies as her mother and now nurse. They were told the chemo would work, but it didn't. The tumor grew. The doctors didn't tell Jennifer and Hannah things were getting worse. Radiation was added to the plan, but by May, Jennifer knew what was happening. She saw it in Hannah's eyes. The end was coming.

Hannah loved the movie "The Fault in Our Stars"—a story about young people with cancer, full of light and grief, humor and heartache. It reminded Jennifer that her daughter, though dying, was still holding on to love and hope in her final days. On August 6, 2020, Hannah passed away. She was surrounded by care—but also by the failures of a system that never stopped to ask why.

After Hannah's death, Jennifer returned briefly to the Cleveland Clinic. She took the oncology nursing exam, knowing in her heart she could make a change, and passed. She pleaded with leadership to consider a functional oncology clinic—to look upstream, to ask better questions. They said no. So, with no backup plan and nothing but her grief and a calling, she walked away. She resigned.

Jennifer went on to found her own practice—Hyperion Functional Medicine—and began to study functional oncology at the cellular and molecular level. She wrote her e-book before she even opened her doors. She built treatment protocols that target the hallmarks of every tumor. She surrounds herself with researchers, nutritionists, and health coaches. She uses off-label pharmaceuticals and research-based supplements to support patients alongside standard care. She has lost only two patients in the years that followed—both of whom were already in advanced chemotherapy with terminal Stage IV breast cancer when they met her.

Today, Jennifer honors Hannah by helping others live. She does not take no for an answer. She looks for what everyone else overlooks. She walks with patients from diagnosis to healing, asking the questions that no one in the system asked her when it mattered most.

Her story reminds us why functional medicine matters. Why advocacy matters. Why listening matters.

And most of all, why healing must begin with humanity.

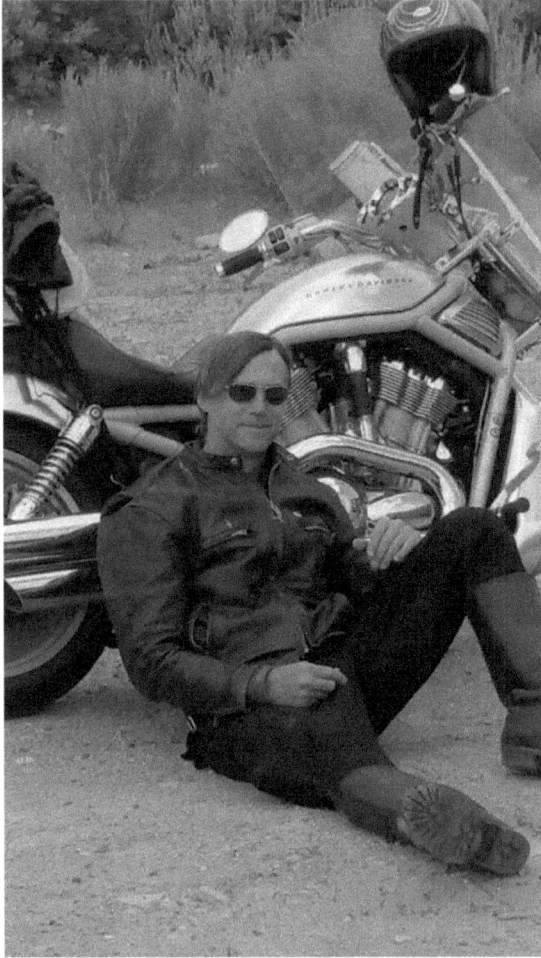

Reid, doing what he loved—riding free, full of life and faith.

Chapter 11

When the System Fails Someone You Love - Reid's Death

When I learned of Reid's cancer diagnosis, I was in shock. Reid was a very private person—he didn't tell any of us he was sick. What we didn't know was that he had a rice-sized lump in his left thigh for many years. About a year before the diagnosis, he noticed it was slowly getting bigger and sought treatment. A local dermatologist, concerned, referred him to an oncologist. Reid was sent to one of the top cancer institutions in the United States—names I won't mention, because it's not about them. What matters is that they made the mistake of cutting into the tumor and leaving positive tumor margins, and under their "watchful" eye, the cancer spread. First to behind his ear; he noticed a strange bump arise there. Then to his lungs.

By the time of his last PET scan before March 2018, a physician told him it was terminal. He had started coughing up blood. They sent him home to get his affairs in order. No hope. No treatment plan. Just time to die.

Reid and my cousin were working on legal cases together at the time and shared an email address. That's how the diagnosis surfaced. A pathology report from the cancer center arrived in the shared inbox. My cousin opened it, confused, and brought it to me. I took one look—and my stomach dropped. I knew immediately it was bad. My cousin, Reid's best friend, was devastated. I had to be the one to tell him Reid might not make it. Then, we had to approach Reid. I begged him to let me help. He agreed, but only on one condition: I wasn't allowed to tell my sister.

It was agonizing. I carried the weight of that secret for nearly six weeks. Finally, when doctors at his first major cancer treatment center told him that chemotherapy would likely do nothing—that it might give him two extra months, at best—he gave me permission. I'll never forget standing in my sister's kitchen as she unloaded the dishwasher. I looked at her, and she just knew. A glass slipped from her hands and shattered. "What's wrong with him?" she asked, clutching her stomach. I told her: "He has cancer. And it's very bad." We both collapsed into tears.

Delivering that kind of news is something I've done countless times as a physician. We're trained to do it. We learn how to say it with empathy, but without feeling. You become numb. You block the emotion so you can function. But this wasn't a patient. This was my family. And the numbness didn't work.

Reid began chemotherapy. For a while, his labs held steady, but the tumors in his lungs grew. More appeared. Each scan worse than the last. They changed his chemo regimen several times, but—just as predicted—nothing worked. No one ever mentioned alternative therapies. Not even for comfort. The doctors only talked about the ineffective drugs: it's all they knew.

By the fall of 2018, they offered him a clinical trial. A brand-new drug. Experimental. Uncertain. I was incredibly reluctant. I'd reviewed the literature, and as a physician, I knew it wouldn't work. I also knew it was risky. At the same time, I was urging Reid to travel out of the country with me to seek alternative care. I'd found Dr. Ralf Kleef in Vienna, Austria who had published cases of advanced sarcoma remission using integrative therapies. Reid, however, was deeply patriotic and a devout Christian. He believed if he was meant to be healed, it would happen in his own country. He enrolled in the trial.

And so, I supported him. Because that's what we're supposed to do as doctors—present information, allow the patient to decide, and support them. Through spring of 2019, Reid took the experimental drug.

His condition rapidly worsened. It was like watching him deteriorate in fast-forward. I can't say definitively that it was the drug, but I know it was.

By May 2019, he was done. No more chemo. No more clinical trials. He was ready to explore alternative options. I wish he'd made that decision earlier. Around that same time, I enrolled in Functional Medicine University. I had watched him be poked, prodded, scanned, and drugged—with no one ever asking how he felt, how he slept, how his soul was holding up. Just numbers. Just CT scans. Just drugs. There had to be another way.

Ironically, I had already been introduced to functional medicine by my sister. Both of us suffered from autoimmune disease. She had reversed her psoriasis through root-cause healing and had been urging me to study functional medicine for years. I hadn't had the time—between motherhood, medical practice, and caring for Reid. But now, I was determined. I completed the two-year program in just seven months, determined to learn all I could, and hoping for an ounce of something that would help.

I dove into the oncology modules first and through my studies, I discovered two oncologists practicing integrative medicine. We met with them virtually—one in Arizona, one in Colorado. They were incredible. They offered us hope and tools that conventional medicine never had. We also found a naturopathic oncologist in Dayton, Ohio—just a few hours away. She became Reid's favorite doctor. She prayed with him at every visit. Her presence brought him peace.

She introduced us to mistletoe therapy. Mistletoe is a botanical treatment used in Europe for decades. It modulates the immune system, improves quality of life, and can slow tumor growth. Reid responded to it beautifully. But by then, we were racing against time.

My only regret is that we didn't start sooner. The doctors knew their drugs wouldn't work. They knew the clinical trial was a shot in the dark. But they pushed it anyway—because it's all they knew. They weren't trained to ask "why." They weren't trained to treat the whole person.

When we told Reid's oncologist we were done—with the trial, the scans, the meds—he looked at us blankly and said, "But he's going to die anyway. Why does it matter?" I was stunned. He didn't say goodbye. He didn't wish Reid well. He just walked out. It wasn't about Reid. It was about the trial.

Reid and I left that appointment and had lunch together. Over lunch, he told me his vision had been off. I assumed cataracts or dry eye from the chemo drugs and promised to examine him. We went our separate ways—he back to Kentucky, me to West Virginia. He never made it home.

For two days, we couldn't find him. Finally, after calling local hospitals, we discovered him in the ICU at the University of Kentucky. He'd had a stroke while waiting at a red light. His brain scans were clear of tumors, but the experimental drug he had taken was known to cause strokes—though the manufacturer didn't list it. I know that's what did it.

Reid was never the same after that. He had to relearn how to walk. He lost vision in one eye. I'm an ophthalmologist, and I couldn't help him. I blamed myself for not recognizing the stroke symptoms sooner. But I realize now—it wasn't my fault. It was the drug. And it was the system.

After the stroke, Reid came to live with me and my sons, ages 6 and 8. He was supposed to stay temporarily—but he never left. For four months, we cared for him as he declined. I lay awake at night listening to him cough up blood, terrified I'd find him dead in the morning. I was helpless.

Then it happened—exactly how I'd imagined. At 5 a.m., my eight-year-old son screamed, "Mommy, Reid needs you!" Reid was gasping for air. His oxygen was maxed out. He'd peed himself from fear. I tried to draw up his morphine with shaking hands. Called 911. My children witnessed every moment. I still remember my youngest hugging Reid and telling him, "It's going to be okay."

I had a clinic full of patients that morning. I was torn between duty and grief. I actually agonized over canceling my day. That's how deeply doctors are conditioned—to keep showing up, no matter what.

Reid had told me how he wanted to die: outside, under the sky. He hated hospitals. But when the firetruck came to take him away, it was the last time he saw our home. He died two days later in the ICU. His lungs were bleeding out. Blood transfusions didn't help. The ventilator kept him comfortable, and before they intubated him, he looked at me and said, "You have three days. Jonah was in the belly of the whale for three days. If I'm still alive and on the ventilator after that, pull the plug." I said, "Okay."

Prior to being intubated, Reid asked to see my sister. I had notified her of his condition, and she was frantically trying to make it there. She walked in just in time. As she ran in, just as the doctors were about to intubate him, she leaned down and kissed his face. They said "I love you" to each other. And Reid got his wish; hers was the last face he saw when his life was coming to an end.

He died the next day. Peacefully, on the ventilator. With all of us by his side.

His hospital room had a massive picture window. I opened the blinds wide. He got his sky.

Later, the funeral home needed a blood family member's consent to release his body. I was his medical power of attorney, but it wasn't enough. I took the phone and explained who I was. The voice on the other end said, "Oh my gosh, Dr. Skeens—it's Nancy. You gave me back my vision. I can see so well now, and I thank you." She was the owner of the funeral home. She came herself. Treated Reid with dignity. I collapsed into tears. It was all so surreal.

Doctors are human, too.

A few days later, she delivered his ashes to me in a beautiful urn—a gift.

No charge.

You never forget what it feels like to hold someone you love in a box.

This is what changed me. This is why I practice differently now.

As I reflect on those final hours with Reid, I would be remiss if I did not acknowledge one individual whose presence made all the difference:

I want to take a moment to express my deepest gratitude to Jamie Spencer, the nurse practitioner who cared for Reid during his final days in the ICU. In those sacred and difficult hours, Jamie provided extraordinary compassion, wisdom, and presence—not only for Reid, but for our entire family. He ensured that Reid passed with dignity, comfort, and peace. For this, I will be forever in his debt. While this book critiques systemic policies regarding scope of practice, it is not a critique of the many dedicated nurse practitioners whose skill and humanity enrich the lives of their patients every day. Jamie embodied the very best of the healing professions, and I honor him here with my whole heart.

In the months that followed Reid's death, I found myself returning to the work of Dr. Ralf Kleef, a visionary integrative oncologist based in Vienna. His landmark 2020 study described a treatment protocol for advanced-stage cancer patients using low-dose checkpoint inhibitors, interleukin-2, mistletoe, and therapeutic hyperthermia. Unlike the high-dose immunotherapy protocols that cause dangerous side effects, Dr. Kleef used lower doses of ipilimumab and nivolumab—just enough to stimulate immune activity without overwhelming the system. He combined this with fever-inducing therapies and immune-supportive infusions.

In his study of 131 patients with Stage IV cancers, including sarcoma, he saw remarkable results: over 30% of patients responded to the treatment, some with complete remission. These were patients conventional medicine had already given up on. And yet under his care, they were healing. He treated the body's terrain, not just the tumor. He looked for the why. His work gave me clarity that our system had missed something fundamental: You cannot heal a person if you do not see them as a whole.

That's why I do things differently now.

While revisiting documents from the time I spent with Reid, I came across an email I had written to a mutual friend of ours. Composed just two days after Reid's passing, it captures my raw and immediate emotions regarding his cancer journey. What follows is that email, preserved in its original form.

Excerpt from Email, November 4th

It is with a heavy heart that I share that Reid passed away peacefully on the morning of Saturday, November 2nd.

Unfortunately, we discovered far too late in his care the work of Dr. Ralf Kleef, an Austrian physician who has successfully treated nearly 200 metastatic sarcoma patients. Trained at MD Anderson and Memorial Sloan Kettering, Dr. Kleef has become recognized internationally as a sarcoma specialist.

I've grown increasingly disillusioned with oncology care in the U.S.-especially when it comes to rare tumors. Reid consulted top sarcoma oncologists at multiple major institutions over two years. Yet, despite different names and affiliations, they all offered the same ineffective drugs, following rigid protocols even when outcomes were poor. The pharmaceutical industry's influence runs deep.

It was a naturopathic oncologist and published author, Dr. Natalie Winters, who finally introduced us to Dr. Kleef. We met with him just a few weeks ago. His center is preparing for a Phase 1 clinical trial for patients exactly like Reid. He has documented cases of sarcoma patients in remission for over a decade-outcomes unheard of in the conventional literature.

His treatment protocol is innovative and measured: low-dose immunotherapy injected directly into lesions (as opposed to the toxic high doses used in the U.S.), checkpoint inhibitors, hyperthermia, IV mistletoe, and high-dose IV vitamin C. I genuinely believe that had we found him a year earlier, we would be telling a very different story.

Reid reminded me of you in many ways. He cherished his alone time. Every summer, he'd take a month off work and ride across the country alone on his motorcycle. He was deeply compassionate-quietly paying each January for a homeless man in his town to stay in a hotel for the month.

He was a public service attorney, a storyteller, a fiercely loyal friend. His life was filled with so many quiet acts of goodness.

Reid lived with me during the final four months of his life. I became his primary caregiver as we planned for our trip to Austria, scheduled for November 18. He had just been cleared by pulmonary rehab to travel without issue. Then, unexpectedly, several tumors in his lungs hemorrhaged, and he passed shortly after.

It is now my mission to document Reid's life and his journey with sarcoma-to tell the truth of what went wrong and to help others avoid the same devastating mistakes. I'm gathering every piece of documentation-messages, correspondence, medical records-so that his voice and experience won't be lost.

It would make a powerful story for you-perhaps even a film. There is, of course, the love story component. My sister and Reid loved each other from the moment they met. Though they tried multiple times to make it work, timing never aligned. Yet it was her face he saw last. And her voice he heard in his final moments, saying "I love you."

I wanted you to know of his passing.

I hope you're doing well.

Heather

The days following Reid's passing felt like a dream I couldn't wake up from. I remember pulling into my garage, numb, and carrying in the bookbag he had with him at the hospital—the same one he had taken in his travels around the world. His reading glasses still stuck out of the front pocket. I hung it on the coat rack by the door, and seven years later, it still hangs there. I've never been able to take it down. I spent most of that day crying, carefully packing up his belongings and moving them to the attic. They've stayed there, untouched. On the way home from the hospital, I stopped by my boys' father's house to pick them up. They had been staying there the last two nights while I was with Reid in the hospital. They were only six and eight at the time. When I pulled up, they came running to the front steps, asking if Reid was coming home. I had to tell them the words I was still struggling to say out loud—Reid died. My eight-year-old broke down crying, screaming "No!" My six-year-old looked up at the sky and whispered, "Reid is with God now, and he is okay." Today, we still talk about Reid. We laugh at the memories, we honor him every November 2nd, on the day of his passing, and we carry him with us.

Reid made me the physician I am, and he taught my children what it means to live—and what it means to let go.

In the quiet after Reid's passing, I found myself asking questions that medicine had never taught me to ask. Questions about why the system failed him, and why my own body was failing me, too. His journey ignited something in me, not just as a physician, but as a human being desperate to understand how we heal. I began to look inward. What I discovered would change the course of my life, my health, and the way I practice medicine.

As I studied functional medicine, I looked at my own signs and symptoms. Years of GI distress, brain fog, itchy skin, autoimmune flares—I had chalked it all up to genetics as conventional medicine had trained me to believe. But through testing, I discovered mold toxicity, celiac disease, adrenal fatigue, and severe nutrient deficiencies. Addressing these root causes put my autoimmune disease into remission, and it has remained there since. I don't suffer from any of these things anymore.

Functional medicine asks why. It doesn't silence symptoms; it solves them. In my studies, I discovered the gut houses 70% of the immune system. I learned how chronic inflammation fuels disease. I studied mistletoe therapy, ozone, hyperbaric oxygen, nutritional protocols. I pursued and obtained a medical cannabis certification because opioids didn't work for Reid—but cannabis did. It relieved his pain, allowed him to sleep, and brought him peace. Cannabis has been villainized, while pharmaceuticals have been glorified. It's absurd. It shouldn't be that hard to find something so ancient and effective.

Reid lived three times longer than expected. He died knowing he was loved, cared for, and finally seen as a whole person. That's what medicine should be.

This chapter is for him. For all the "Reids." For every doctor who has loved someone and found themselves powerless.

And for every patient who gave something back to us when we needed it most—thank you.

The Doctors Who Remembered Him

Following Reid's passing, I made it a point to personally notify all the physicians who had cared for him throughout his journey. Out of all the doctors involved, only two reached back out to offer their condolences—both integrative medical practitioners—reminding me that even in a broken system, there are still healers who lead with their hearts. Reid's favorite physician, Dr. Vanessa Edwards, ND of Dayton, Ohio, wrote, *"He was very special and loved by so many, including me… I find consolation in knowing we will spend eternity together."* Her warmth and faith reflected everything Reid cherished in a caregiver. Dr. Ralf Kleef, MD, an internationally respected integrative oncologist in Vienna, Austria—whom we had consulted with via Skype and were scheduled to visit before Reid passed—also reached out. He wrote, *"Remember, that love cannot die… You will be connected forever."*

Tragically, Dr. Kleef himself would pass away in 2021 from COVID-19, at just 60 years old. A visionary in the field of cancer immunotherapy and fever therapy, his legacy lives on in the lives of the patients he treated and the physicians he mentored. He left behind a profound legacy in the world of integrative oncology. Dr. Gurdev Parmar, a fellow physician and close friend, honored his passing by writing:

"Ralf became a close friend of Helen Coley-Nauts, daughter of William B. Coley, MD–the father of Cancer Immunotherapy... This relationship inspired Ralf's focus on hyperthermia and fever therapy in cancer treatment."

Dr. Parmar went on to say, *"Ralf, you will be dearly missed. You have left a huge hole in the field of integrative cancer care... Your loss will be felt by both patients and doctors alike. You have left us all way too early, my friend. May you rest in peace."*

Both Dr. Edwards and Dr. Kleef showed me what medicine looks like when compassion leads, and connection is not lost. They treated Reid not just as a patient, or a diagnosis, but as a soul. Their words, their presence, and their humanity remain etched in my memory and left a profound mark on me—and theirs are the kind of hearts I hope more doctors will learn to model. They embodied what medicine can be at its best: human, heartfelt, and whole.

Chapter 12

Fragmented Medicine: How the System Breaks Doctors the Same Way It Breaks Patients

Medical school doesn't teach root-cause healing. It doesn't teach whole person healing. It teaches symptom management. It teaches drugs.

From the moment doctors enter training, they are courted by pharmaceutical companies—lunches, presentations, influence. What we're not taught is how to reverse disease. We learn almost nothing about nutrition. Nothing about lifestyle. Nothing about prevention. We don't learn to ask why. We learn to prescribe.

We are trained in algorithms and symptom suppression. And those of us who dare to challenge this system—who step outside the pharmaceutical model to advocate for food as medicine, for emotional healing, for root-cause testing—are often punished. Some lose licenses. Others are publicly discredited. But a shift is happening. Medicine is waking up. More physicians are recognizing the limitations of conventional care. We are turning toward functional medicine, holistic approaches, and whole-person healing.

Patients are awakening to change as well. It is daily now that I have multiple patients inquiring of how they may address the root of their issues. I am asked about what vitamins they should take to help slow or reverse the progression of their cataracts and keep their retina healthy. I am told they are making dietary changes and exercising. I am asked "why" has a problem developed and not simply, "what medication will fix it."

Medical training must evolve. We must begin to train doctors on root cause medicine, nutrition, and lifestyle changes. We must reduce the crushing debt that comes with becoming a physician. We must lessen administrative burdens and insurance interference so that doctors can spend their time doing what they were trained to do—care for patients, not battle red tape. We must prioritize physician mental health and restore autonomy. This isn't optional. It's necessary if we want to preserve the heart of medicine.

The Truth About Physician Exploitation: The Modern-Day Slavery of Medicine

The exploitation of doctors begins in residency, where they are expected to work inhumane hours for unlivable wages. It is beyond comprehension that a physician with 12 years of education, six-figure debt, and life-or-death responsibilities is paid less than a front desk receptionist. Yet doctors are groomed to believe that financial security is greedy, while hospital executives and insurance companies rake in billions. Why are doctors, nurses, veterans, and first responders—the very people who sacrifice their lives for society—the most undervalued, underpaid, and overworked professionals?

The public assumes doctors are rich, but here's the reality: Physicians graduate with an average of $250,000+ in debt and spend a decade in training before they even start making a livable wage. Many will spend years repaying loans, and by the time they establish themselves, malpractice insurance, disability insurance, licensing fees, and professional expenses eat away at their earnings. Doctors are also the only professionals expected to work for free. A lawyer charges for a consultation, but a physician is expected to provide free medical advice. A financial planner bills for an email response, yet a doctor must answer messages at all hours for free or risk a lawsuit.

Physicians are akin to professional athletes—expected to sacrifice their bodies and minds for their careers—yet unlike an athlete, they don't have multimillion-dollar contracts, sponsorships, or structured retirement plans. Instead, most doctors work themselves into exhaustion and die shortly after retirement, their bodies and minds broken by the very career they dedicated their lives to. If doctors are expected to sacrifice and push their bodies like professional athletes, then why aren't they paid and protected like them? Why as a society, are our priorities so askew?

Physicians are conditioned to go to work sick, ignore exhaustion, pain, and emotional trauma, perform at peak levels despite chronic stress, PTSD, and physical deterioration.

The physiological toll of medicine is staggering.

Physicians suffer from chronic stress-induced neurodegeneration, leading to memory loss, brain fog, and emotional instability. The constant fight-or-flight response damages the hippocampus, impairing cognitive function over time. Long work hours and relentless stress result in sky-high rates of heart disease, hypertension, and metabolic syndrome. Doctors have some of the highest rates of heart attacks and strokes—a direct consequence of the cortisol overload they endure daily.

Medicine also accelerates aging and disease. Gray hair, skin inflammation, gut disorders, and autoimmune conditions are all exacerbated by chronic stress. Many physicians struggle with chronic pain, fatigue, and adrenal burnout, yet they are expected to push through, or risk being labeled weak.

The cruel irony? The people responsible for keeping society healthy are among the sickest, most burned-out population.

So, what can be done? The future of medicine depends on addressing the deep systemic issues that have pushed physicians to their breaking point. Reducing administrative burdens would allow doctors to focus on what they were trained to do—care for patients—rather than drowning in paperwork and insurance battles. Reforming medical education costs and alleviating the crushing debt burden would ensure that the best and brightest continue to enter the profession without the fear of financial ruin. Prioritizing physician mental health and work-life balance would help prevent burnout, depression, and the tragic loss of talented doctors who can no longer endure the pressure. Restoring physician autonomy by reducing insurance interference would empower doctors to make medical decisions based on what is best for their patients, not on what is most profitable for corporations. These are not small changes; they require a fundamental shift in how we view and value the people who dedicate their lives to healing others. But if we fail to act, medicine will no longer be a noble calling—it will become a cautionary tale of how a once-revered profession was driven into the ground by a system that refused to change.

The Medical System Is Designed to Keep Patients Sick

Medical school does not teach doctors to practice functional medicine. We are trained to benefit the pharmaceutical industry, not to heal patients. From the moment we enter medical training, we are bombarded by pharmaceutical company representatives. They sponsor grand rounds, bring lunch to our meetings, and ensure that we know exactly which drugs to prescribe for which conditions.

What we are not taught is how to help patients prevent disease or reverse chronic illness through diet, lifestyle, and environmental interventions. Shockingly, medical students receive almost no formal education in nutrition—despite the fact that diet is one of the most critical factors in disease prevention and healing.

We are not taught how to identify nutrient deficiencies, test for metabolic imbalances, or counsel patients on food as medicine. Instead, we are trained to write prescriptions, perpetuating a system in which chronic disease is managed—but never cured. Those of us who speak out about this reality risk losing our medical licenses.

Many pioneering physicians who have advocated for root-cause medicine have been ostracized from the medical community for going against the status quo. But the truth is, medicine is evolving. More and more physicians are recognizing the limitations of conventional medicine and turning to a functional, holistic approach that prioritizes true healing rather than endless disease management.

Like any profession, medicine is not without its small percentage of individuals whose actions tarnish the reputation of the many. Stories of insurance fraud, unethical billing practices, and unnecessary procedures make headlines, painting a distorted picture of the profession. There are reports of physicians abusing prescription drugs, overprescribing narcotics, or engaging in misconduct reinforcing negative stereotypes. However, what is rarely highlighted are the countless acts of integrity, sacrifice, and dedication that physicians demonstrate daily. The narrative surrounding medicine is often skewed, focusing on scandals and malpractice rather than the millions of lives saved, the selfless hours worked, and the unwavering commitment doctors have to their patients.

While accountability is crucial, it is equally important to recognize that the vast majority of physicians enter this field with a deep sense of duty, compassion, and a desire to heal. The system breaks us. Doctors do not enter medicine broken—we are rigorously screened before even stepping foot into medical school. A history of drug abuse, addiction, or mental health struggles can disqualify a candidate before they ever have a chance. Yet despite beginning their journey full of passion and purpose, many doctors do not emerge the same way.

It is not the profession itself that destroys them; it is the system. The relentless sleepless nights, the reliance on stimulants just to stay awake, the neglect of basic self-care, and the gradual erosion of physical and mental well-being take their toll. The gut microbiome is disrupted, leading to depression, anxiety, and ADHD. Doctors, in their desperate attempt to survive an inhumane system, become dependent on the very prescription drugs they were once trained to manage responsibly. A system that demands superhuman performance while offering no room for human weakness pushes them to the breaking point.

At the same time, physicians are robbed financially, emotionally, and psychologically. They are burdened with massive debt and systemically underpaid for the intensity and years of sacrifice required to reach their position. They struggle to find fair compensation, and some, out of sheer desperation, make unethical or regrettable decisions just to survive. While not excusable, these actions cannot be separated from the years of dehumanization, bullying, and exploitation physicians endure from administrators, hospital systems, insurance companies, and sometimes even their own patients.

Doctors experience burnout, imposter syndrome, and suicidal ideation at alarming rates, yet society refuses to acknowledge the systemic abuse they suffer. Veterans, police officers, and teachers—those in professions that serve and sacrifice—are rightly granted early retirement and financial security in recognition of their contributions. Yet no such relief exists for doctors. Instead, they are expected to work until they die, trapped in a system that demands everything from them yet gives nothing in return. The expectation is clear: Physicians must give their lives, their youth, their mental well-being—and when they are no longer useful, they are discarded.

This is the reality of medicine today. And it is why the system must change.

The System Was Never Built to Heal

When students enter medical school, they do see people as whole. They carry within them a pure, almost sacred belief that healing means treating the entirety of a person—mind, body, and spirit. But that vision doesn't last. Because from day one, medical education begins to teach us otherwise. We are trained to compartmentalize. To reduce human beings into systems, symptoms, and organs. Psychiatry for the mind. Gastroenterology for the gut. Dermatology for the skin. Ophthalmology for the eyes. Each piece separated, siloed, studied, and treated in isolation as if the soul doesn't bind it all together.

We are taught to treat the parts, not the person. And in doing so, we begin to forget that the body is not a machine—it is a living, breathing ecosystem, rich with interdependence.

But what's even more tragic is this: The system doesn't just do this to the patient. It does the exact same thing to the physician.

Doctors, too, are broken into pieces.

Doctors enter medicine because they want to heal, to serve, and to make a difference in people's lives. But the current system is pushing them to the brink emotionally, physically, and financially. If our mind begins to crack under the weight of trauma or exhaustion, we are given a diagnosis and offered a drug. Depression? Try an SSRI. Anxiety? Here's a benzodiazepine. Suicidal thoughts? Hospitalize, medicate, and move on. But no one asks why. No one looks at the root cause. The chronic sleep deprivation. The moral injury. The loss of autonomy. The soul-crushing bureaucracy that replaces purpose with productivity metrics. No one treats the system that created our suffering—they just treat the symptoms.

When our bodies begin to falter—our backs give out from standing in the OR for 12 hours straight, our adrenal glands collapse from years of fight-or-flight, our guts revolt against processed cafeteria food and relentless stress—we are handed pain pills, antacids, and stimulants. We're patched up and sent back to the front lines. As if the problem is within us, not the machine we're trapped inside.

The healthcare system dissects its own healers in the same way it trains us to dissect our patients. It refuses to see us as whole.

We are not just surgeons. Not just data entry clerks. Not just prescribers. We are artists, parents, poets, athletes, musicians, caregivers. But the system strips that away. It values only the part of us that bills. The part that shows up for a 7 a.m. surgery. The part that codes correctly and sees more than 40 patients a day. All other parts are ignored—or worse, penalized.

And so, just like our patients, we become fragmented. Reduced. Disconnected from ourselves. And when a doctor is treated like a machine, is it any wonder that burnout, depression, addiction, and suicide are so rampant?

We are not broken people. We are people broken by a system.

If we want to heal our patients, we must first heal the system. And to do that, we must stop pretending that healing lives in a prescription pad. Healing lives in wholeness. In connection. In being seen.

Medicine has forgotten this.

But we don't have to.

If we do not address these issues, we will continue losing our best doctors, and patients will suffer as a result. The physician shortage is already worsening, and the healthcare industry cannot function without those willing to dedicate their lives to medicine.

Chapter 13

Fixing a Broken System: Solutions to Physician Burnout and the Mental Health Crisis

Physician burnout is not an unavoidable byproduct of practicing medicine—it is the result of systemic failures that push doctors beyond their limits. If we do not act now, we will continue to lose physicians at an alarming rate, further worsening the growing doctor shortage and reducing the quality of patient care. The good news is that change is possible. We can rebuild medicine into a profession that respects and sustains its healers. But doing so requires real reforms across multiple areas of the healthcare landscape.

One of the most urgent steps is to address physician mental health. Doctors are suffering in silence, fearful that seeking help will lead to career consequences. Many state medical boards and credentialing bodies still include intrusive mental health questions on licensing applications, discouraging physicians from disclosing their struggles with depression or anxiety. Removing these questions is crucial—no doctor should have to risk their livelihood to receive care. Hospitals and training programs must also provide confidential mental health resources, including designated advocates who can guide physicians to safe and anonymous support. More importantly, we must normalize mental health conversations in medicine. When respected leaders speak openly about their own experiences, the culture of silence begins to break.

Work-hour reform is another essential pillar of change. Medical trainees and attending physicians are routinely overworked to dangerous levels, often enduring shifts of 24 hours or longer without sleep. These conditions lead to burnout, medical errors, and deteriorating physical and mental health. It's not enough to have work-hour restrictions on paper—they must be enforced. No doctor should be forced to sacrifice their own health or family life to practice medicine. Flexible scheduling, increased staffing, and limits on shift length are proven solutions already implemented in countries like Norway and the Netherlands, where physicians work fewer hours and patient outcomes are better.

Equally damaging is the administrative burden created by insurance companies. Physicians are forced to spend precious hours fighting for prior authorizations, submitting excessive documentation, and appealing denials—all while patient care suffers. We need a healthcare system that values medical judgment over bureaucracy. Eliminating unnecessary prior authorization hurdles, increasing reimbursement for quality, patient-centered care, and reducing red tape will give doctors back the time and energy to focus on healing.

Financial reform is long overdue. Physicians often begin their careers with more than $250,000 in debt, and yet many face stagnating salaries and rising overhead costs. Medical students should not have to choose between their calling and financial survival. Expanding loan forgiveness for those serving in underserved areas, increasing reimbursement rates for Medicare and Medicaid patients, and offering tax credits to independent practices are actionable steps to ensure that medicine remains a sustainable profession. Some states have already created repayment programs for rural physicians—but we need federal-level reform to make an impact on a national scale.

Perhaps the greatest challenge is reclaiming control of healthcare from those who do not practice it. Hospital administrators, insurance executives, and policymakers often dictate the rules of modern medicine, prioritizing profits over patient care. Physicians must be empowered to lead again. Hospitals and medical organizations need more doctors—not corporate managers—in decision-making roles. Independent practices must be protected and encouraged, giving physicians autonomy over how they care for their patients. Legislative advocacy is key here. Some states have already banned non-compete clauses for physicians, freeing them from toxic environments. More collective action is needed.

We must also prioritize physician work-life balance. For too long, the culture of medicine has glorified self-sacrifice. But this mindset is toxic and unsustainable. Doctors should not have to choose between being good physicians and having a fulfilling personal life. Medical systems should support part-time and flexible options, paid parental leave, family care resources, and wellness training built into education and practice. Some hospitals have already introduced on-site childcare and mandatory wellness days—this must become the standard, not the exception.

Doctors shouldn't have to choose between their careers and their well-being. They shouldn't have to fight insurance companies for every treatment or sacrifice their health for the sake of others. But fixing this broken system will require a multi-pronged approach: legislative action, cultural transformation within medicine, and a demand from both physicians and patients for lasting change. It's time to stop telling doctors to be "resilient" and start repairing the system that is breaking them.

The fight for a better future doesn't rest on doctors alone. Everyone—physicians, patients, and policymakers—has a role to play. If you're a doctor, speak up. Support mental health initiatives and advocate for work-hour reform. If you're a patient, demand better healthcare. Support reforms that prioritize the well-being of doctors, because a healthy physician provides better care. If you're a policymaker, listen. Work alongside physicians to craft a healthcare system that serves both patients and providers with dignity.

Physicians are not expendable. Yet the current system treats them as if they are. If we do nothing, we will continue losing our most passionate and skilled doctors—not because they no longer love medicine, but because the system has crushed their ability to practice it safely. This is not just a physician crisis—it is a crisis for every patient, every family, and the future of healthcare itself. The time for passive acceptance is over. Change begins now.

To the physicians reading this: you are the backbone of healthcare. You carry the knowledge, the skill, and the compassion that saves lives. But you are also human. Take back control of your profession. Speak up when conditions are unsafe. Seek help when you are struggling. Do not suffer in silence. Consider unionizing. Join advocacy groups that push for physician-led care. Get involved in policy. Walk away from toxic workplaces if necessary. Explore models like concierge medicine, telehealth, or solo practice if they bring you more peace and purpose. Reclaim your voice. The future of medicine belongs to those who fight for it.

To the policymakers: your decisions directly affect the health of our doctors and, in turn, the well-being of our entire population. Remove mental health disclosure requirements. Enforce humane work-hour limits. Regulate insurance companies and reduce the red tape that stands between a doctor and their patient. Support student loan forgiveness and better compensation. Invest in the independent practices that prioritize quality care over corporate quotas. Every law you write that uplifts doctors will ripple outward to benefit patients.

To the patients: this is your fight, too. You deserve better. Demand lawmakers who care about physician wellness. Speak out against long wait times, poor access, and declining quality of care—because these are symptoms of a crumbling physician workforce. Support physician-led clinics. Advocate for price transparency. And most of all, support the doctors who support you. They are fighting for your life while barely holding on to theirs.

Medicine should be about healing, not harm. It should be a place where doctors can thrive—not just survive. But that future won't create itself. It will take collective effort. Physicians must demand better. Policymakers must listen. Patients must rise up. Because what's at stake isn't just the future of doctors—it's the future of care itself.

Let's fix this. Not someday. Now.

Real-World Success Stories: Physician-Led Initiatives and Healthcare Reforms That Work

While physician burnout and the healthcare crisis may seem overwhelming, there are real examples of progress happening right now. Across the country—and around the world—doctors, advocacy groups, and innovative policymakers are stepping up to reclaim the integrity of medicine. They're working to improve physician well-being and create better outcomes for patients. These stories offer not only hope but a clear roadmap forward.

One of the most promising developments has been the growth of Direct Primary Care (DPC) in the United States. Frustrated by the red tape of insurance-driven medicine, physicians are leaving traditional corporate models to open DPC practices. These practices eliminate insurance altogether and operate on a monthly membership basis-much like a gym. Patients pay a set monthly fee, usually between $50 and $100, and in return receive unlimited visits, no copays, and direct access to their doctor. Doctors in DPC settings typically manage smaller patient panels—around 600 rather than the traditional 2,500—and are able to spend more time with each patient, often 30 to 60 minutes per visit. The benefits are significant: reduced overhead, less bureaucracy, and most importantly, dramatically lower rates of physician burnout. A shining example of this model's success is Epiphany Health in Florida, founded by Dr. Lee Gross. In 2010, Dr. Gross left the insurance-based system and established his own DPC clinic, where patients enjoy transparent pricing and preventative care, and hospitalizations have dropped as a result. His clinic proves that when doctors reclaim their autonomy, everyone benefits.

Work-hour reforms are another area showing real promise. In Sweden, New Zealand, and even some forward-thinking hospitals in the U.S., healthcare systems have been experimenting with the four-day workweek for physicians. The results have been remarkable: Doctors are less burned out, more engaged, and make fewer errors. In a two-year trial conducted at a hospital in Gothenburg, Sweden, physicians worked six-hour shifts across four days instead of five. Doctors reported significantly improved work-life balance, enhanced mental health, and increased energy during patient visits. Even patient wait times dropped, as productivity per hour rose. Hospitals also saved money by reducing turnover and recruitment costs. These results clearly show that providing physicians with humane schedules doesn't compromise care—it enhances it.

Another breakthrough is occurring in the fight against prior authorizations. These time-consuming hurdles imposed by insurance companies have long been a source of frustration for doctors and delay for patients. But some states have stepped up with real solutions. Texas made headlines in 2021 when it passed the Gold Card Law, allowing doctors with a 90% or higher approval rate on prior authorizations to bypass the process entirely. This not only frees physicians from mountains of paperwork but also ensures patients receive timely treatments. States like Kentucky and Washington are beginning to follow suit. These reforms are proof that smart legislation can protect both doctors and patients, reducing stress while improving care.

Beyond policy, grassroots physician advocacy is also driving change. Organizations like The Physicians Foundation are actively lobbying for physician well-being, publishing annual reports on burnout, and advocating for regulatory reform. The Physician Moms Group (PMG), with over 100,000 members, has become a powerful force for parental leave policies and peer support in medicine. The DPC Alliance continues to help doctors transition to independent, insurance-free practices that prioritize meaningful patient relationships. These groups are not waiting for permission—they are leading the way.

After leaving Cleveland Clinic's Functional Medicine Center, Dr. Shah founded her own private practice. "I needed autonomy," she explains. "I needed to be at my kid's baseball game and still care for patients the way I was trained to. So, I built a model that worked for me." Her practice now serves women and children using root-cause medicine, and she continues to advocate for smarter pediatric and environmental health approaches. "Patients are sick. They're coming in with chronic illness that conventional medicine isn't solving. Functional medicine gives us another lens—and it works."

The truth is change is already happening—but it must accelerate. The success of direct care models, work-hour reforms, and physician-led legislation offers a clear path forward. What we need now is expansion. More states must pass physician-friendly laws. More hospitals must adopt humane schedules. More physicians must reclaim their independence and autonomy.

The system is not beyond repair. These stories prove that a better future is possible—and that future begins with the collective action of physicians, policymakers, and patients alike. Medicine is worth saving. And the doctors who dedicate their lives to it are worth saving, too.

Chapter 14

Bellasee™: A Movement Rooted in Physician Liberation

Bellasee™ is a system designed to emancipate physicians from the chains of healthcare slavery. Bellasee™ isn't just a franchise. It is a movement. A movement built by doctors, for doctors—specifically those who have felt betrayed by the system they gave their lives to. Bellasee™ gives power back to the physician. It restores autonomy, equity, and dignity to the practice of medicine.

At its core, Bellasee™ is about reclaiming the doctor-patient relationship—removing insurance interference, reducing hospital control, and bringing medicine back into the hands of the people who actually practice it. It is a model designed to protect the healer as much as it heals the patient.

A New Model for Women in Medicine

Medicine, as it exists today, is still structured for men—particularly white men—leaving women and underrepresented minorities at a severe disadvantage. Work schedules, leadership pipelines, pay structures, and systemic biases continue to push women and minority physicians out of the profession. The reality is that the traditional medical system was never built for us, and it is failing doctors and patients alike. The solution is not just in acknowledging the problem but in creating a system that allows all physicians to thrive. That's where Bellasee™ comes in. Bellasee™ is not just an ophthalmology franchise—it is a revolution in how medicine is practiced, structured, and sustained for the future. By shifting power away from corporate hospital systems, insurance companies, and male-dominated leadership boards, Bellasee™ provides physicians—especially women and minority doctors—with the autonomy, financial security, and work-life balance they deserve.

Bellasee™, while optimal for both male and female doctors, was initially designed with women physicians in mind. Traditional medicine still functions on outdated models—schedules built for men who don't carry the weight of caregiving. Women in medicine are penalized for needing balance. They're forced to choose between being a mother and being a surgeon.

At Bellasee™, we reject that false choice. Our model allows flexible schedules, part-time options without penalty, and total physician autonomy. Female doctors become owners—not employees. They create their own schedules, build their own practices, and finally achieve the balance that has long been denied to them.

Work-Life Balance: A System That Works for Women Physicians

Women physicians are burning out at record rates, largely because medical work schedules are still designed for men who are not expected to carry primary caregiving responsibilities. Mothers in medicine are often forced to choose between career advancement and their families, and traditional medicine punishes doctors for wanting balance.

Bellasee™ reverses this narrative by offering flexible schedules, physician-owned autonomy, and clinic hours that align with real life. No longer are doctors required to work 80-hour hospital shifts or adhere to rigid structures that make raising a family nearly impossible. Bellasee™ also supports female physicians in entrepreneurship, shifting them from employees to owners and allowing them to build their own schedules without fear of financial instability. Part-time work options are encouraged without career penalties—something that is nearly unheard of in hospital-based medicine. Bellasee™ creates an environment where women don't have to choose between being great doctors and great mothers.

Leadership and Ownership: Giving Women and Minority Physicians Power

Despite making up over 50% of medical school students, women hold only 18% of leadership roles in medicine, with even fewer positions going to Black and Latino physicians. The hierarchy of hospital leadership remains a "boys' club," where men control promotions, salaries, and career opportunities. Bellasee™ flips this system upside down. It offers physician ownership, eliminating the need for doctors to wait for male-dominated hospital boards to decide their fate. Women and minority doctors become business leaders as franchise owners, transforming them from employees into CEOs of their own practices. Financial independence follows naturally, without the gender-based pay gaps that dominate traditional medicine. Bellasee™ puts power back in the hands of physicians, particularly those who have been historically excluded from leadership.

Diversity in Medicine: More Opportunities for Black and Latino Physicians

The lack of diversity in medicine remains staggering. Only 5% of U.S. doctors are Black, and only 6% are Hispanic despite these groups making up a much larger percentage of the population. Minority medical students face greater financial barriers to entering medicine, and patients in underserved communities struggle to find doctors who look like them.

Real change requires more than policy—it requires people. It requires someone in the room who sees what others miss. It requires doctors who recognize that talent isn't always reflected in test scores, and that mentorship can be the difference between a thriving physician and a lost one. One of the most powerful stories I've heard came from a Black academic cardiologist who served as a residency program director. What he shared with me will stay with me forever.

He Was in the Room

I spoke with a Black academic cardiologist—one who prefers to remain anonymous—whose journey and integrity have shaped more lives than he'll ever know. For the purposes of this book, we'll call him Dr. Julian West.

Julian was not only a practicing cardiologist with a research lab but also served as a residency program director in a prominent academic medical center in the Midwest. His leadership wasn't just administrative—it was transformational. He was nominated by the house staff, not because he sought power, but because he earned their trust. And during his five years in that role, he changed the face of medicine in his program.

He told me about a student—Black, bright, and passionate—whose board scores were, on paper, disqualifying. His resume was strong, his recommendations glowing, but without someone advocating for him, he likely would have been overlooked. Julian insisted they bring him in for an interview. He saw something in this student that couldn't be measured by test scores. That student went on to become one of the best residents they had—ultimately rising to become chief resident in that institution. Being named chief resident is a prestigious honor in medicine, signifying exceptional leadership, clinical excellence, and the highest level of trust from faculty in a highly competitive environment.

All because Julian was in the room.

But Julian's story isn't just about one student—it's about a pattern. During his time in leadership, minority enrollment rose. When he left, it dropped. Not because the pipeline dried up, but because no one remained in the room to ensure Black and Brown students got a fair shot.

He shared how, in interviews, Black candidates were often critiqued for being "nervous"—a coded excuse not given to White applicants. He had to speak up and say, "Everyone's nervous." And once those minority students were accepted, they became victims of what he called "benign neglect." They didn't get meaningful mentorship. Their evaluations were vague. If a White student struggled, someone stepped in. If a Black student struggled, no one noticed until it was too late.

Julian believes in accountability—but also in understanding the burden of culture. "We are taught we must work twice as hard. That we cannot ask for help. That to show weakness is to be dismissed." That burden leads many minority physicians to burn out in silence, without ever asking for the help they so desperately need. He wants to change that.

One of the most moving things he told me was about the patients. How many times he walked into a room and was met with surprise. Some patients assumed he couldn't be the doctor. A few even refused his care. But when he walked into the room of a Black patient, their entire face would light up. In him, they saw hope. Safety. Trust. They saw someone who looked like them—and they knew they'd be heard.

"Black excellence in medicine isn't a unicorn," he said. "We exist."

He advocates for more diverse leadership—not just for symbolic purposes, but for real outcomes. Hiring managers, admissions boards, and faculty panels must include underrepresented voices; else, implicit bias will continue to shape who gets through the door. He calls this "The P.I.E. Principle" for minority advancement: Productivity, Image, and Exposure. To succeed, you need all three. You can't just work hard in silence. You have to show your value and be seen.

And to medical schools and hospitals across the country, he offers a challenge: If you want diverse talent, go find it. Reach beyond the default hiring pool. Compete for it. Because if you don't, schools like Harvard will—and they'll get the best.

To young minority doctors, he says: "Find mentors who believe in you, even if they don't look like you." Representation matters, but so does genuine advocacy. And when you find success, don't be afraid to become the advocate for others. You might be the only one in the room—but sometimes, one is all it takes.

Stories like Julian's remind us that representation isn't just symbolic—it's life-altering. Having a single advocate in a position of power can open doors that would otherwise remain closed. At Bellasee™, we aim to build more rooms where every voice is heard, where mentorship is intentional, and where no qualified physician is ever overlooked because of the color of their skin or the weight of systemic bias.

Bellasee™ actively increases minority representation by mentoring and supporting underrepresented doctors. Bellasee™ helps minority physicians own their practices, gain leadership roles, and break the cycle of exclusion. Bellasee™ directly increases minority-owned medical practices, providing more equitable healthcare access for diverse populations. It gives doctors a chance to own their practice, build generational wealth, and serve the communities they come from—without having to wait for a seat at someone else's table.

Cash-Based, Patient-Focused: Ending the Insurance Trap

Insurance has hijacked the doctor-patient relationship. Physicians spend more time filling out paperwork than treating people. Bellasee™ lessens this burden. Our offerings for direct-care and cash-based models eliminate third-party interference. We train physicians in the art of offering cash payments to patients. We teach them how to find additional streams of income outside of direct patient care, so they may not feel pressure to only see patients for revenue generation. We provide them an education in business and entrepreneurship.

Doctors spend more time with patients, offer transparent pricing, and regain control of how care is delivered. Meanwhile, patients benefit from real relationships with their doctors.

Generational Wealth and Financial Freedom for Doctors

In traditional medicine, doctors are employees. They don't own their time. They don't own their earnings. And they certainly don't own their practice. Bellasee™ changes that.

Bellasee™ gives physicians equity. Ownership. The ability to build long-term financial freedom. Women and minority doctors no longer have to rely on male-dominated hospital boards for raises or promotions. They become CEOs of their own lives and practices.

From Burnout to Balance

Doctors today are suffering. Burnout. Brain fog. Broken marriages. Health crises. This is the price of practicing medicine inside a broken system.

Bellasee™ was built to end that cycle. Our model prioritizes work-life balance. Clinic hours that make sense. Autonomy over schedules. No more 100-hour weeks or missed birthdays.

We built a system where doctors can thrive, not just survive.

Residency is modern-day slavery. Doctors with 12 years of education make less than minimum wage while carrying hundreds of thousands in debt. They work 80 to 120 hours per week. They collapse from exhaustion, suffer from PTSD, and develop chronic illness—and we call it a "rite of passage."

Bellasee™: A Revolution in Medicine

Bellasee™ is more than a solution. It's a stand. A stand against exploitation. A stand for empowerment. Medicine grinds doctors down. But Bellasee™ builds them back up. We know what it means to feel exploited. And we've built a model that flips the script. No more asking for permission to rest. No more begging administrators to approve a vacation. Bellasee™ lets doctors live again. Bellasee™ is the blueprint for what medicine can—and should be.

We've heard enough about broken systems. It's time to build a new one.

Bellasee™ is the way forward. For doctors. For patients. For medicine itself.

Final Thoughts: Bellasee™ as a Blueprint for the Future of Medicine

Medicine should reflect the people it serves. Doctors should have control over their own careers. Wealth should be accessible to all physicians, not just those who fit the traditional mold. Bellasee™ offers physicians a way out of the broken system, a chance to double or triple their income, and most importantly, a work-life balance that does not require sacrificing career success.

Physicians are slaves to a system that was never designed to support them. It's time to break free.

Bellasee™: Not Just a Franchise

Medicine is broken—not just flawed but fundamentally rigged against the very people who dedicate their lives to healing others. Physicians are trapped in a system that demands their bodies, minds, and financial stability, yet offers little in return.

No other profession demands so much, costs so much, and compensates so little. No other career path requires over a decade of training, only to pay its trainees less than minimum wage. No other industry forces its workers into a life of physical and emotional sacrifice, with no structured plan for rest, retirement, or recovery.

And yet doctors are expected to work for free, be grateful for their suffering, and never ask for more. If they dare advocate for fair compensation or work-life balance, they are shamed as greedy, selfish, or ungrateful. Society throws millions of dollars at professional athletes, influencers, and entertainment moguls, while the physicians who literally keep humanity alive are treated as expendable resources.

Bellasee™ is a doctor-led solution to an industry built to exploit physicians. It offers doctors a way out, a path to financial freedom, and a return to autonomy—without sacrificing patient care.

Bellasee™ isn't just about building a business. It's about taking back medicine. It allows physicians to double or triple their income without working themselves into the ground, regain work-life balance, and break free from the abusive cycle of hospital and insurance control while still practicing medicine on their own terms.

Bellasee™ was created to break the cycle of physician exploitation and build a sustainable, financially empowering, doctor-owned future. Doctors should not have to choose between practicing medicine and having a life. Doctors should not be the most overworked, underpaid professionals in America. Doctors should own their careers—not be owned by the system. Bellasee™ is not just a business. It's an option for fair pay, work-life balance, physician empowerment, and a breaking free from a system that does not value its healers.

The medical industry will not change on its own. The people who run it profit from physician suffering. Change will only happen when doctors take back control. Bellasee™ is the way out. The way forward. The way to reclaim medicine.

Chapter 15

Final Thoughts

Doctors, you must recognize that you are worth far more than the healthcare system leads you to believe. You have dedicated years—sometimes decades—to mastering your craft, and yet the system often treats you as replaceable. It's time to rise above this mindset. But before you can reclaim your autonomy, you must first believe in yourself. You must cultivate confidence in your own value, skills, and purpose. Once you do this, you will command the respect you deserve from colleagues, nurses, patients, and administrators. And if they do not offer that respect, you will not be burdened by it—you will know that their lack of regard reflects them, not you.

As physicians, we are the leaders of our healthcare teams. In moments of exhaustion—when surgeries run hours longer than expected, when headaches pound, when hunger gnaws, and when frustration builds—it is crucial to remain composed. Your team looks to you for direction. If you maintain resilience and professionalism, they will follow your lead. This is not to say that burnout and exhaustion should be accepted as normal; they shouldn't be. But in the midst of a tough situation, anger and outbursts solve nothing. Instead, endure the challenge with grace, then take proactive steps to prevent it from recurring.

For instance, if your surgical schedule consistently runs over, address it—not with frustration in the moment, but with clarity and conviction afterward. If you prefer your OR days to end by 2 p.m. because six straight hours under the microscope is your limit, enforce that boundary. Some physicians may handle longer days, while others need less. The key is knowing your own limits and ensuring they are respected.

If overbooking leads to late evenings in the OR, don't take it out on your team or patients. Instead, have a direct conversation with your scheduler and ensure it doesn't happen again. You are responsible for your own well-being, and if something is not working for you, change it. Do not accept being a victim of a broken system.

Many doctors feel trapped, believing that working in academic medicine or large private group practices is the only path forward. These environments strip us of control—governing our schedules, our patient care decisions, and even the number of hours we must work. But this is not true autonomy, and this is not true life. We are among the most intelligent professionals on the planet, expected to absorb immense amounts of knowledge in a short time. Yet we are not given even the most basic business education in medical school. Have you ever stopped to ask why? Have you considered that this omission is intentional? That it is designed to keep us dependent, to keep us subservient to administrators and corporations who dictate how we practice medicine?

The healthcare system is structured to take advantage of us. It is time to break free.

Bellasee™ is an opportunity for doctors to reclaim their autonomy, to restore work-life balance, to own their own practices, and to care for their patients the way they see fit. It is a community where we can learn from one another and support each other in becoming the best versions of ourselves—both professionally and personally.

We must ask ourselves: Why do we allow people with no medical knowledge to sit in corporate offices and dictate how we care for our patients? Why do we permit private equity firms to buy our practices, convincing us that they are more qualified to run them? If a corporation sees your practice as valuable, that means it has worth—so why would you give it up? If they want it, why don't you?

Doctors, it is time to take back control. Not just for ourselves, but for our patients, our profession, and the future of healthcare. This is your life—your one and only life. Live it on your terms.

Join the Bellasee™ Movement
Reclaiming Medicine. Together.

Bellasee™ isn't just a clinic. It's not just a franchise. It's a movement—built by doctors, for doctors, with one unifying goal: to restore what medicine was always meant to be.

Physicians: You deserve autonomy, financial freedom, and a life that honors your calling without breaking your body. Patients: You deserve care that sees your whole person, not just your lab results.

We are building a future where doctors own their work, patients trust their providers, and healing happens without interference from bureaucracy and broken systems.

Bellasee™ is that future.

- Visit www.bellasee.com
- Learn how to start your own Bellasee™ practice—or find a Bellasee™ provider near you
- Contact us to bring Bellasee™ to your community.
- Are you a physician outside of ophthalmology who's ready to reclaim your autonomy? If you're interested in starting a Bellasee™ clinic within your specialty, we'd love to hear from you. Contact us to explore how the Bellasee™ model can be adapted to fit your field and empower your practice.

References

Chapter 2

1. Starr, P. (1982). *The social transformation of American medicine*. Basic Books.

2. Porter, R. (1997). *The greatest benefit to mankind: A medical history of humanity from antiquity to the present*. W.W. Norton & Company.

3. Lad, V. (2002). *Textbook of Ayurveda: Fundamental principles (Vol. 1)*. The Ayurvedic Press.

4. Dharmananda, S. (2000). *Chinese medicine and modern science: Herbal treatment perspectives*. Institute for Traditional Medicine and Preventive Health Care.

5. Zhao, Z., & Chen, H. (2011). *Pharmacology and applications of Chinese materia medica*. Science Press.

6. Weil, A. (2004). *Health and healing: The philosophy of integrative medicine and holistic healing*. Houghton Mifflin Harcourt.

7. World Health Organization. (2019). *WHO global report on traditional and complementary medicine 2019*. World Health Organization.

8. Sneader, W. (2005). *Drug discovery: A history*. John Wiley & Sons.

9. Swann, J. P. (1988). *Academic scientists and the pharmaceutical industry: Cooperative research in twentieth-century America*. Johns Hopkins University Press.

10. Flexner, A. (1910). *Medical education in the United States and Canada: A report to the Carnegie Foundation for the Advancement of Teaching*. The Carnegie Foundation.

11. Wallace, A. R. (2009). *The untold story of Rockefeller medicine.* Skyhorse Publishing.

12. Gawande, A. (2002). *Complications: A surgeon's notes on an imperfect science.* Picador.

13. Berenson, A. (2021). *Pandemia: How coronavirus hysteria took over our government, rights, and lives.* Regnery Publishing.

14. Offit, P. A. (2021). *You bet your life: From blood transfusions to mass vaccination, the long and risky history of medical innovation.* Basic Books.

15. Caplan, A. L., & Redman, B. K. (2020). *Bioethics and the COVID-19 pandemic.* Springer.

16. Breggin, P., & Breggin, G. (2021). *COVID-19 and the global predators: We are the prey.* Lake Edge Press.

17. Senger, J. (2022). *The war on ivermectin: The medicine that saved millions and could have ended the COVID pandemic.* Skyhorse Publishing.

18. Gøtzsche, P. C. (2013). *Deadly medicines and organised crime: How big pharma has corrupted healthcare.* Radcliffe Publishing.

19. Berenson, A. (2021). *Pandemia: How coronavirus hysteria took over our government, rights, and lives.* Regnery Publishing.

20. Offit, P. A. (2021). *You bet your life: From blood transfusions to mass vaccination, the long and risky history of medical innovation.* Basic Books.

21. Caplan, A. L., & Redman, B. K. (2020). *Bioethics and the COVID-19 pandemic.* Springer.

22. Breggin, P., & Breggin, G. (2021). *COVID-19 and the global predators: We are the prey.* Lake Edge Press.

23. Centers for Medicare & Medicaid Services. (2021). *Omnibus COVID-19 health care staff vaccination interim final rule with comment period.* U.S. Department of Health and Human Services. Available from https://www.cms.gov

24. Gold, S. (2022). *I Do Not Consent: My Fight Against Medical Cancel Culture.* Bombardier Books.

25. Kennedy, R. F. Jr. (2021). *The Real Anthony Fauci: Bill Gates, Big Pharma, and the Global War on Democracy and Public Health.* Skyhorse Publishing.

26. Association of American Medical Colleges. (2021). *The complexities of physician supply and demand: Projections from 2019 to 2034.* AAMC. Available from https://www.aamc.org

27. Senger, J. (2022). *The war on ivermectin: The medicine that saved millions and could have ended the COVID pandemic.* Skyhorse Publishing.

28. Jabbour, S., Torres, M. F., & Dubovy, S. R. (2020). *Corneal transplant rejection associated with influenza vaccination: Case report and literature review. Cornea, 39*(5), 663–665. https://doi.org/10.1097/ICO.0000000000002200

29. Phylactou, M., Li, J. P. O., & Larkin, D. F. P. (2021). *Acute corneal transplant rejection after COVID-19 vaccination. Eye, 35,* 289–291. https://doi.org/10.1038/s41433-02101630-3

30. Brennen, J. S., Simon, F. M., Howard, P. N., & Nielsen, R. K. (2020). *Types, sources, and claims of COVID-19 misinformation.* Reuters Institute. https://reutersinstitute.politics.ox.ac.uk/types-sources-and-claims-covid-19-misinformation

31. Ball, P. (2021). *The lightning-fast quest for COVID vaccines-and what it means for other diseases.* Nature, 589(7840), 16–18. https://doi.org/10.1038/d41586-020-03626-1

Chapter 3

1. Association of American Medical Colleges. (2024). *AAMC FACTS: Table A-1. U.S. medical school applications and matriculants by school, state of legal residence, and sex, 2023–2024*. AAMC. https://www.aamc.org/data-reports/studentsresidents/report/facts

2. Association of American Medical Colleges. (2024). *About the MCAT® exam*. AAMC. https://students-residents.aamc.org/applying-medical-school/taking-mcat-exam/about-mcat-exam

3. Association of American Medical Colleges. (1999). *Medical school applicants and matriculants data, 1998*. Washington, DC: AAMC.

4. Association of American Medical Colleges. (2024). *Table A-1: U.S. medical school applications and matriculants by school, state of legal residence, and sex, 2023-2024*. Retrieved from https://www.aamc.org/data-reports

5. Kirch, D. G., & Vernon, D. J. (2020). *Transformation of the U.S. medical education system: A new framework for the future of medical training*. Academic Medicine Publishing.

6. Association of American Medical Colleges. (2023). *Medical school enrollment reaches a new high*. Retrieved from https://www.aamc.org/news/medical-school-enrollment-reaches-new-high

7. Association of American Medical Colleges. (2021). *The complexities of physician supply and demand: Projections from 2019 to 2034*. AAMC.

8. Lee, P. P., Jackson, C. A., & Relles, D. A. (2020). *Workforce projections for ophthalmology: A national perspective*. American Academy of Ophthalmology.

Chapter 4

1. Wikipedia contributors. (n.d.). *Medical school in the United States*. Wikipedia. Retrieved April 19, 2025, from https://en.wikipedia.org/wiki/Medical_school_in_the_United_States

2. Physicians Thrive. (2024). *Physician compensation report*. Retrieved from https://physiciansthrive.com

3. CompHealth. (2024). *The state of physician burnout and retention*. Retrieved from https://comphealth.com

4. Med School Insiders. (2023). *Residency dropout rates and burnout explained*. Retrieved from https://medschoolinsiders.com

5. Med School Insiders. (2023). *Understanding the medical training process: Challenges, burnout, and residency dropouts*. Retrieved from https://medschoolinsiders.com

6. MedSchoolCoach. (2023). *The reality of medical school and physician burnout: Training, debt, and mental health*. Retrieved from https://medschoolcoach.com

Chapter 5

1. Sierles, F. S., Brodkey, A. C., Cleary, L. M., McCurdy, F. A., Mintz, M., Frank, J., & Woodard, J. L. (2005). Medical students' exposure to and attitudes about drug company interactions: A national survey. JAMA, 294(9), 1034–1042.

2. Wazana, A. (2000). Physicians and the pharmaceutical industry: Is a gift ever just a gift? JAMA, 283(3), 373–380.

3. Grande, D., Frosch, D. L., Perkins, A. W., & Kahn, B. E. (2009). Effect of exposure to small pharmaceutical promotional items on treatment preferences. Archives of Internal Medicine, 169(9), 887–893.

4. Brennan, T. A., Rothman, D. J., Blank, L., Blumenthal, D., Chimonas, S. C., Cohen, J. J., & Smelser, N. (2006). Health industry practices that create conflicts of interest: A policy proposal for academic medical centers. JAMA, 295(4), 429–433.

5. Yeh, J. S., Franklin, J. M., Avorn, J., Landon, J., & Kesselheim, A. S. (2016). Association of industry payments to physicians with prescription behavior. JAMA Internal Medicine, 176(8), 1114–1122.

6. Institute of Medicine. (2009). Conflict of interest in medical research, education, and practice. Washington, DC: The National Academies Press.

7. Centers for Disease Control and Prevention. (2014). Insufficient sleep is a public health epidemic. Retrieved April 2014 from https://www.cdc.gov/features/dssleep/

8. Institute of Medicine. (2006). Sleep disorders and sleep deprivation: An unmet public health problem. Washington, DC: The National Academies Press.

9. Schernhammer, E. S., & Colditz, G. A. (2004). Suicide rates among physicians: A quantitative and gender assessment (meta-analysis). American Journal of Psychiatry, 161(12), 2295–2302.

10. The stories of Dr. Sarah L., Dr. Mark R., Dr. Emily T., and Dr. James P. are composites drawn from multiple physician interviews and real-life cases shared during confidential discussions, anonymized for privacy.

11. Clance, P. R., & Imes, S. A. (1978). The impostor phenomenon in high achieving women: Dynamics and therapeutic intervention. Psychotherapy: Theory, Research & Practice, 15(3), 241–247.

12. Gottlieb, M., Chung, A., Battaglioli, N., Sebok-Syer, S., & Kalantari, A. (2020). Impostor syndrome among physicians and physicians-in-training: A scoping review. Medical Education, 54(2), 116–124.

13. Cutter, C. (2023). America's New Millionaire Class: Plumbers and HVAC Entrepreneurs. The Wall Street Journal. Retrieved from https://www.wsj.com/articles/ americas-new-millionaire-class-plumbers-and-hvac-entrepreneurs-117a0b19

Chapter 6

1. Association of American Medical Colleges. (2023). *Financial trends in U.S. medical schools: FY2023 report.* AAMC.

2. American Hospital Association. (2023). *AHA Hospital Statistics: 2023 edition.* Health Forum.

3. Wikipedia. (2023). *Madeline Bell (executive).* Retrieved from https://en.wikipedia.org/wiki/Madeline_Bell_(executive)

4. Wikipedia. (2023). *Ascension (healthcare system).* Retrieved from https://en.wikipedia.org/wiki/Ascension_(healthcare_system)

5. Paddock Post. (2023). *Executive compensation at UPMC (University of Pittsburgh Medical Center).* Retrieved from https://paddockpost.com/2023/06/20/executive-compensation-at-upmc/

6. U.S. Congress. (2020). *Coronavirus Aid, Relief, and Economic Security (CARES) Act.* Public Law No. 116-136. U.S. Government Publishing Office.

7. Mathematica & National Academy for State Health Policy. (2022). *Despite increased labor costs, hospitals saw record profits during the pandemic.* Mathematica. Retrieved from

https://www.mathematica.org/news/despite-increased-labor-costs-nationally-hospitals-saw-record-profits-during-pandemic

8. Whaley, C. M., Briscombe, B., & DeYoreo, M. (2022). *How hospitals fared financially during the COVID-19 pandemic.* JAMA Health Forum. RAND Corporation. Retrieved from https://www.rand.org/pubs/external_publications/EP70180.html

9. Tsai, T. C., Jha, A. K., & Orav, E. J. (2021). *Disparities in allocation of COVID-19 relief funding among hospitals.* JAMA Network Open, 4(12), e2138271. https://pmc.ncbi.nlm.nih.gov/articles/PMC8727033/

10. Urban Institute. (n.d.). *Health and hospital expenditures.* Urban Institute. https://www.urban.org/policy-centers/cross-center-initiatives/state-and-local-finance-initiative/state-and-local-backgrounders/health-and-hospital-expenditures

Chapter 7

1. Tucker, M. E. (2024, March 6). *Former UCLA doctor receives $1.4 million in gender discrimination case.* Medscape. Retrieved from https://www.medscape.com/viewarticle/former-ucla-doctor-receives-14-million-gender-discrimination-2024a10009ei

2. Roberts, L. M. (2019, November). *For women in business, beauty is a liability.* Harvard Business Review. https://hbr.org/2019/11/for-women-in-business-beauty-is-a-liability

3. Wikipedia contributors. (n.d.). *Physical attractiveness stereotype.* Wikipedia. Retrieved April 11, 2025, from https://en.wikipedia.org/wiki/Physical_attractiveness_stereotype

4. Her Culture Staff. (2018, October 18). *Unequal burden: Dress code expectations on women in the workforce.* Her Culture. https://www.herculture.org/blog/2018/10/18/unequal-burden-dress-code-expectations-on-women-in-the-workforce

5. Wilson, E. (2024, April). *Pretty privilege: The ugly truth about appearance discrimination.* Labor and Employment Law Insights. https://www.laborandemploymentlawinsights.com/2024/04/pretty-privilege-the-ugly-truth-about-appearance-discrimination

6. Heilman, M. E., & Saruwatari, L. R. (1979). When beauty is beastly: The effects of appearance-based sex stereotyping on evaluations of job applicants for managerial and non-managerial jobs. *Organizational Behavior and Human Performance, 23*(3), 360–372. https://doi.org/10.1016/0030-5073(79)90003-5

7. Chamorro-Premuzic, T. (2019, November 12). For women in business, beauty is a liability. *Harvard Business Review.* Retrieved from https://hbr.org/2019/11/for-women-in-business-beauty-is-a-liability

8. Williams, J. C. (2021). Beauty and the bias: How good looks can work against women in academia. *Women in Higher Education.* Retrieved from https://www.wihe.com/article-details/122/beauty-and-the-bias/

9. Torres, A. (2018, October 18). Unequal burden: Dress code expectations on women in the workforce. *Her Culture.* Retrieved from https://www.herculture.org/blog/2018/10/18/unequal-burden-dress-code expectations-on-women-in-the-workforce

10. Association of American Medical Colleges. (2022). *Diversity in the physician workforce: Facts and figures.* Retrieved from https://www.aamc.org

11. Jena, A. B., Olenski, A. R., & Blumenthal, D. M. (2021). *Sex differences in physician salary in US public medical schools. JAMA Internal Medicine, 181*(2), 230-238.

12. National Academy of Medicine. (2023). *Women in medicine: Progress, barriers, and solutions.* Retrieved from https://nam.edu

13. Williams, D. R., & Cooper, L. A. (2019). *Reducing racial inequities in health: Using what we already know to take action. Health Affairs, 38*(10), 1671-1680.

14. Tsugawa, Y., Jena, A. B., Orav, E. J., Blumenthal, D. M., & Jha, A. K. (2017). *Age and sex of physicians and patient mortality in the United States: Observational study. BMJ, 357,* j1797.

15. Rotenstein, L. S., Sinsky, C. A., & Jena, A. B. (2021). *Gender pay gaps in medicine: Not only a matter of time.* National Academy of Medicine. https://doi.org/10.31478/202110b

Chapter 8

1. Stack, L. (2024, February 13). *Former Intermountain CEO Dr. Marc Harrison shot and killed in Utah; suspect had history of grievances with healthcare system. The Salt Lake Tribune.* https://www.sltrib.com/news/2024/02/13/former-intermountain-ceo-dr-marc

Chapter 9

1. Buerhaus, P. I., Skinner, L. E., Auerbach, D. I., & Staiger, D. O. (2021). Implications of the rapid growth of the nurse practitioner workforce in the US. Health Affairs, 39(2), 273–279. https://doi.org/10.1377/hlthaff.2020.00686

2. U.S. Bureau of Labor Statistics. (2022). Occupational Outlook Handbook: Nurse Anesthetists, Nurse Midwives, and Nurse Practitioners. U.S. Department of Labor. https://

www.bls.gov/ooh/healthcare/nurse-anesthetists-nurse-midwives-and-nurse-practitioners.htm

3. American Medical Association. (2021). AMA defends physician-led care as essential to high-quality patient outcomes. https://www.ama-assn.org/press-center/press-releases/ama-defends-physician-led-care-essential-high-quality-patient-outcomes

4. General Medical Council (UK). (2022). Investigation into patient death highlights risk of inadequate training among physician associates.

5. National Conference of State Legislatures. (2024). Optometry scope of practice expansion legislation. Retrieved from https://www.ncsl.org/health/optometry-scope-of-practice-expansion-legislation

6. Tan, J., Wang, A., & Gregory, L. (2019). Delayed referrals in ophthalmology: A UK-based case series and review. British Journal of Ophthalmology, 103(5), 630–635.

7. Fong, G. H., Kheradmand, A., & Malik, A. (2014). Diagnostic delays in referral to ophthalmology: A retrospective study of visual outcomes. British Journal of Ophthalmology, 98(12), 1684–1689. https://doi.org/10.1136/bjophthalmol-2013-304754

8. American Academy of Family Physicians. (n.d.). Understanding nurse practitioner and physician assistant scope of practice. Retrieved from https://www.aafp.org/family-physician/practice-and-career/managing-your-practice/team-based-care/nurse-practitioner-physician-assistant-scope-education.html

9. American Medical Association. (n.d.). *Scope of Practice.* Retrieved from https://www.ama-assn.org/practice-management/scope-practice

10. Gulland, A. (2024, December 17). Ban physician associates from seeing NHS patients one-to-one, says RCP. The Guardian. Retrieved from https://www.theguardian.com/society/2024/dec/17/ban-physician-associates-from-seeing-nhs-patients-one-to-one-says-rcp

11. Hooker, R. S., & Muchow, A. N. (2023). The changing employment of physicians, nurse practitioners, and physician assistants. Journal of the American Association of Nurse Practitioners, 35(8), 590–598. https://doi.org/10.1097/JXX.0000000000000754

12. Patel, S. Y., & Mehrotra, A. (2023). A fourth of U.S. health visits now delivered by non-physicians. Harvard Medical School News. Retrieved from https://www.ama-assn.org/practice-management/scope-practice

Chapter 11

1. Parmar, G. (2021, December 6). *Dr. Ralf Kleef – 1961–2021: Integrative cancer care pioneer remembered.* Integrated Health Clinic. Retrieved from https://www.integratedhealthclinic.com/dr-ralf-kleef-1961-2021/

Chapter 13

1. Direct Primary Care Coalition. (2023). *A guide to direct primary care: How physicians are reclaiming autonomy and restoring the doctor-patient relationship.* Washington, DC: DPC Alliance Publishing.

2. Gross, L. (2022). *Epiphany Health: A direct primary care success story.* Sarasota, FL: Independent Physician Press.

3. The Physicians Foundation. (2023). *America's physicians: A survey on burnout, mental health, and the future of medicine.* Charlotte, NC: The Physicians Foundation.

4. Physician Moms Group. (2021). *Stronger together: How women physicians are transforming healthcare from the inside out*. PMG Publishing.

5. DPC Alliance. (2022). *Breaking free from the system: A step-by-step guide to launching a direct care practice*. Washington, DC: DPC Alliance Press.

6. Swedish National Health Board. (2020). *Healthcare on four days: Lessons from work-hour reform in Gothenburg hospitals*. Stockholm, Sweden: Health Workforce Innovation Series.

7. Texas Medical Association. (2021). *The Gold Card Law: Legislative victories in healthcare reform*. Austin, TX: TMA Policy Press.

www.ingramcontent.com/pod-product-compliance
Lightning Source LLC
Chambersburg PA
CBHW052113030426
42335CB00025B/2970